On My Feet Again

JENNIFER FRENCH

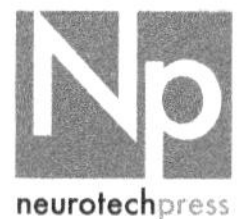

ISBN 978-0-9882342-0-8

Neurotech Press
461 Second St. #124
San Francisco, CA 94107
415 546 1259
415 358 4264 fax
www.neurotechreports.com

For my husband, Tim, who is
My biggest critic,
My toughest therapist,
My loudest voice of reason, and
My dearest friend
With love

Contents

Foreword

by P. Hunter Peckham

I first met Jen French early on during her participation as a research subject—really a test pilot—in our research program. I was the Director of the Functional Electrical Stimulation Center where the research was being conducted and I was told that I should meet her because we had a common interest in sailing. Nothing brings people together like a common love—and for us it was sailing. So it was that I met one of the strongest and most courageous people that I have had the privilege to be around and to work with.

People who choose to participate in human research truly are test pilots. They take upon themselves, possibly for no personal gain, the risks associated with being a pioneer—going where no one or only few have gone before. Although risks versus benefits are carefully evaluated by regulatory bodies before any study can be undertaken—and researchers carefully document those risks and potential benefits—it is still a journey into the unknown for those who decide to participate. In this case, Jen was to become one of the early pioneers evaluating an implanted electrical stimulation device intended to assist her in standing. The possible risks included infection, rejection of the device by the body, and failure to perform the standing function as intended. These test pilots are not frivolous; they are most careful in asking critical questions and evaluating their own personal choices of the potential outcome for them. But they also assess selflessly their contribution to the greater good—to people like them who have sustained similar injuries and may benefit from their contribution even if they themselves do not. They give of their time—and of their body—and journey into the unknown for a greater good to society.

Jen's story is remarkable in every respect. After a life-changing snowboarding accident, which instantaneously took her from an avid outdoor sports enthusiast to wheelchair dependency, she fought back to find the resources that would again enable her independence. That is how our paths crossed, as she looked for research that was ready for prime time to assist her in achieving her goals. For Jen, her participation in the research has enabled her to gain significant capacity to stand and walk, even walking down the aisle at her wedding. She has gone on to have an advanced device implanted, providing even greater function. Only she can say how many of her goals have been achieved, but suffice it to say that every test pilot wants to test the limits of how far they can push the envelope. They always strive for a higher goal.

I would not want to sail competitively against Jen. She is meticulous, calculating, and fearless. She understands the rules of the game, and puts together an unbeatable game plan. You want her on your boat—on your team—she is a winner. And this is the best part for me. We *are* on the same team! And the sport is not a sport at all—it is a mission. And that mission is to ensure that people who have sustained spinal cord injury will always have access to this life-altering implantable stimulation technology.

What began as two sailors talking has become a deep relationship of two people with this common goal. For many with spinal cord injury, this technology offers the best near-term solution for restoration of critical body functions, and to fall short of this goal would be to shortchange thousands of people of key benefits for their health and independence.

Our society is indebted to pioneers like Jen who have the courage to live their convictions, to put themselves on the line, and to work tirelessly to provide a better life for an entire class of disabled people. Jen's willingness to "put herself out there," to be the best that she can be, to challenge herself in every dimension—whether it be competitive sailing or advancement of research—is truly an example of the greatest spirit of mankind.

Acknowledgments

In this book, I've mentioned members of the research team including the surgeons, the engineers, and the therapists. The small team that interacted with me on a daily basis is key to the value of the research. Dr. Ron Triolo is the principal investigator, lead engineer, and maestro of the research team. At times he would pace the floors and at other times he knew how to step aside and let his talented team do their work. He is the brains behind the system that I enjoy today. In the words of a post-doctoral student of his, "Ron is a god of biomedical engineering."

Along with this close research team, there are engineers, like Mike Miller, Stephanie Nogan Bailey, Dawn Lissy, Tina Vrabec, and Jim Uhlir, who are great troubleshooters and translators of engineering lingo. The administrators who dealt with my needs ,like Jeanne Teeter (may she rest in peace), Mary Buckett, Julie Jacono, Laura Polacek, Cathy Naples, and Cheryl Dudek, showed a lot of patience. The doctoral candidates that worked in this project have come and gone over the years, like Sahana, Kofi, and the illustrious Dr. Fisher. The full team of surgeons are some of the most talented in their field with a bedside manner and a sense of humor: Dr. John "Chip" Davis, Dr. James Anderson, Dr. Harry Hoyen, Dr. Gilles Pinault, and Dr. Kutaiba Tabbaa. You have given me the J-Lo butt. The team of nurses: Ruth, Debbie, Mary Beth, Mary Anne, Nancy, and Cathy (who exercised with me) plus Jeanne and Barb gave exceptional care like I've never experienced and would join in sing-alongs from the Muppets and Disney. Because of Barb, I will always know the words to "I Never Go to Work," and will continue to work on my arm wrestling abilities. The therapists in the program probably had the hardest job: dealing with me on every visit. They are talented and truly led the research team to customize a great system. Carol Bieri (may she rest in peace) and Lori Rohde were my cat-loving friends who could always fill the time with another cat story. To Lisa Lombardo, I hope you are impressed.

These are only a few of the research team who touched me. In reality, there is an army of people working on developing this device from the Cleveland FES Center and the Advanced Platforms Technology Center.

There are also the hidden heroes. I've been fortunate to have an incredible support network. My husband, Tim, has sacrificed so much to help me from surgery recovery to functional use. He has become harder on me than the therapist, but I love it. My in-laws, Betty and Joe, are loyal cat-sitters and help with the cleaning while I'm away. My sister Chris and her family have hosted me in their home for the many visits to Cleveland with countless meals and scheduling arrangements. My father, in the early days, would drive and sometimes just accompany me to the lab. His inquisitiveness always kept the conversation flowing. My previous employer, PC Connection, was supportive of me participating in the research and was flexible with my rehabilitation and work schedules.

This book wouldn't be complete without recognizing my Mom. What a trooper; meeting me at the airport in wee-hours of the morning, driving me between hospitals and laboratories, waiting while I have secret squirrel meetings and tests, and pitching in when the research team needs a hand. And the cookies! The research team will forever be spoiled by my mom's cookies. Over the course of time, she has become a member of the research team. She is a true hidden hero.

The research projects that I was able to participate in would not have been possible without the support of the funding agencies that believed in the concept and allowed the research team to make it a reality. The Rehabilitation Research and Development Service of the U.S. Department of Veteran Affairs has been a long time supporter of this research. Yes, these projects are partially funded by the VA. Although I am not a veteran, being a participant in a VA sponsored program is one way that I can give back to our wounded warriors living with spinal cord injuries. One day, they will benefit from the discoveries and assistive technologies resulting from this research. Support for the development and implementation of my systems were also provided by the Office of Orphan Product Development (OOPD) of the U.S. Food and Drug Administration (FDA), the National Institute of Biomedical Imaging and Bioengineering (NIBIB) of the National Institutes of Health (NIH), the Clinical and Translational Science Collaborative (CTSC) at Case Western Reserve University and the Cleveland Clinic Foundation funded by the National Center for Research Resources (NCRR), a component of the National Institutes of Health and NIH roadmap for Medical Research. Generous institutional support was provided by Case Western Reserve University, MetroHealth Medical Center, and the Louis Stokes Cleveland Department of Veterans Affairs Medical Center. Additional support was provided by the Neural Prosthesis Program of the National Institutes of Neurological Diseases and Stroke (NINDS) of the NIH.

This book is an acknowledgment of the commitment that these funding agencies have made to advance the science and clinical translation of lower extremity neuroprostheses for standing, walking, and seated function after spinal cord injuries. The contents of this book are solely the responsibility of the author and do not represent the official views of any of these agencies.

There is another team of people who believed in me and the need to improve access to neurotechnology. Neurotech Network was founded in 2005 as a nonprofit organization to improve education and increase access to neurotechnology for persons with impairments. Jim Cavuoto is my encouragement to keep the organization moving forward even in the toughest times. Jack Gardner and Mary Buckett gave me invaluable advice. Hunter Peckham is my kick in the pants motivator and sailing friend. Without their support and guidance, Neurotech Network would never exist.

Finally, this book can't be closed without thanking all the readers and followers of this journey. The messages of encouragement, gracious cheers and heart-felt notes have helped me along the way. I hope this has helped to build an understanding of the human experience and the required commitments of clinical trials. I am not the only one to participate in the exciting world of scientific development, nor will I be the last. This is one small contribution to the evolution of technology and the progress to improve life for people living with spinal cord injury.

Thank you for getting me back on my feet again.

Chapter 1: Life Before Injury

Stepping out onto the front porch of our historic New England colonial home, you could hear the frozen snow crackle under my feet as I descended down the steps to the street. It was a classic mid-winter morning in New Hampshire.

The Last Morning Run

I was out for my pre-dawn run. In fact, at that time of year, the entire morning routine is before sunrise. The air is frigid. Despite my neck warmer, I could see every breath in the air. My breath was comfortingly warm.

I flipped on my Sony Walkman and started the morning ritual run through the neighborhood. On this run I would be accompanied by the 80's tune, "Everybody Wants to Rule the World," by Tears for Fears. Running and music are my formula of clearing your mind and preparing for the hectic day ahead. Up the steep hill to the top of the neighborhood I go and the thighs are starting to burn. I barely notice since my mind has now wandered onto other things.

The year was 1998. The dotcom bubble had not yet burst the U.S. economy. I was happy with my decision to move a few years earlier, switching careers from finance to technology. It was almost like moving from the old-boys club to the latest fashion scene. Frustrated with the pace of the finance business at the time, joining a dotcom was like reconnecting with my peers. Dotcoms were abundant and workaholics were pushing to be the first at what was coming next. We were all striving to be innovators on the latest Internet frontier. I was in my mid-twenties, and joining the company PC Connection was the move I would make and the buzz that would motivate me.

Living in Manchester, New Hampshire, my live-in boyfriend at the time, Tim, and I rented the bottom half of a classic colonial. It had plenty of room for two people and was in a good location on the north side of the city. We weren't ready to commit to owning a home. Hell, we weren't ready to commit to each other!

Tim and I met while I was still in college. We both worked for the same company at the Norwood Airport in Massachusetts. After surviving two years of living away from each other, we figured our relationship would survive. We found our home in upper New England and pursued our careers. We lived by the motto "Work hard, play hard." We barely saw each other during the work week. On weekends, it was up early to enjoy the outdoor activity of choice for the season. During winter, it was snowboarding or snow shoeing and the ideal playground was in our backyard within the White and Green Mountains of New Hampshire and Vermont.

Life was good. Life was vibrant. Nothing could go wrong.

Slippery Slope

PC Connection, the small company that I had joined a few years earlier, went public in March 1998. Leading up to that event, it was a circus. Working weekends and late nights was the norm to get this feat accomplished. Now that the event was behind us and the NASDAQ was the exchange to watch, it was time to take some time off.

For several years, we had a tradition of joining a group of friends at a ski resort. We would rent a slope-side house that slept a dozen people but stuff an extra half dozen in too. It was a weekend of skiing/snowboarding all day and playing poker and drinking beer all night. Over the course of the weekend, we would finish a keg, or two and smoke way too many cigarettes.

We typically took this weekend in March during the height of spring ski season. The days were longer and the crowds at the resorts were not as bad. This year, Tim and I were in charge of getting the kegs. Being the beer snobs and being in southern

New England, we decided to swing by the Long Trail brewery to get our choice beer. Sure, it was a little pricey, but I had dotcom stock inching its way up in value. We would take off work on Friday to arrive at the mountain late morning. Move in and get at least a half day of boarding in.

As planned, we had a great half day to finish it off with a beer in the lodge before heading back to the slope side house. Tapping the Long Trail kegs, the beer began to flow for the weekend. Soon the never-ending poker game commenced. For this Friday—Friday, March 13th—there was a full moon.

It was a perfect opportunity for our traditional "midnight run." For the run, the most sober of the group would take the pickup truck to the base of the mountain while a group of daredevils would suit-up, grab our boards or skis, and head for the slopes. This time, Tim was encouraging me not to go.

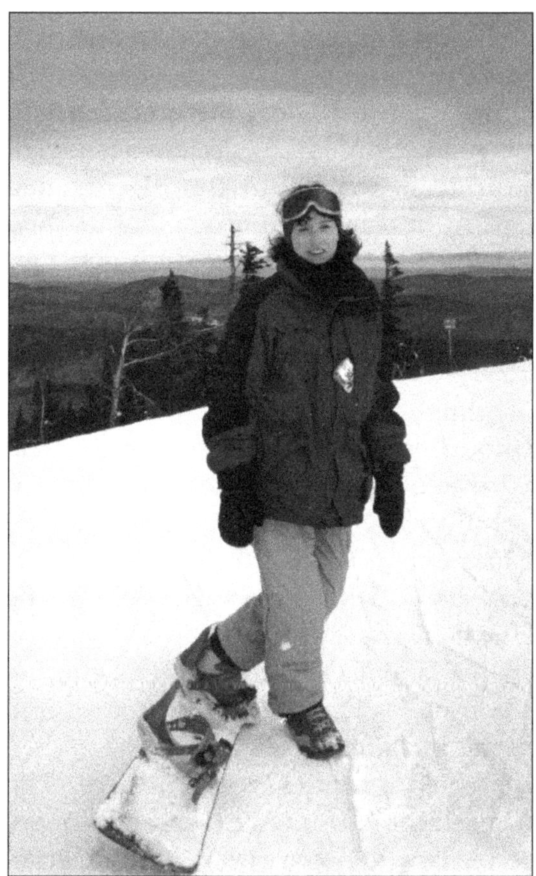

Me and my snowboard

"Come on. You've done this before. I have a bad feeling about this," he prodded.

Being persistent, I pushed back. "This is the perfect time with a full moon. Come on, don't be chicken. It'll be fun."

And back and forth we went, as I pulled on my snowboarding gear. Finally realizing that he wasn't going to stop me, Tim suited up and joined me on the slope.

Just as expected, the

full moon was high in the sky. The moonlight made the ski slopes glow in the darkness of the forest. Sitting in the middle of the slope and strapping on our snowboards, I had to sit back and enjoy the view. It was one of those images; the ones that a camera can never catch but will be etched in your mind forever.

"Okay, let's go!"

The group headed down the mountain. I held back, wanting to get my space among the group—and also to enjoy the serenity. The ride was icy and it became harder and harder to dig in the edge of my board. Nearing the bottom, I took a break and sat down with my board and feet in front of me. Fighting the slippery ice was getting too hard, so I decided to work the edges to get the powdery snow. Something didn't feel right, but I didn't know what it was. I took a look up at the moon, got up and proceeded on the final stretch to the bottom.

Working the edges for powder seemed to work and I began to relax. But along with that relaxation came carelessness. I hit a patch of ice and slid off the trail. Unable to stop, I careened down a 40-foot embankment. At first it was just snow, but then came the army of trees. My body bounced off one, then another. It was happening in slow motion, but in a flash it was over. Lying helpless in the snow, I looked up to the moon in the sky.

"Help."

That was the last thing I remembered.

Down at the base of the mountain, the gang gathered up. Tim was already down there and was impatiently waiting for me. After a while, his irritability changed to dire concern. He headed back up the trail on foot. Far enough away from the rattle of the others, he heard a weak cry. Looking over the side of the trail, he spotted me face down in the snow off the side of the embankment. Sliding down the snow until he reached me, he knew something was really wrong. Tim's instinct kicked in and he offered verbal comfort to me but didn't touch me.

Feeling the urgency to get help as quickly as possible, Tim started crawling back up the embankment. The same slippery slope that landed me in the trees was now preventing Tim from getting back to the trail. Crawling and digging in his boots, he finally made it back to the trail. Sprinting down the mountain, he went to the lodge searching for a telephone. There was no one outside but some people inside the lodge.

Seeing a mad man banging on the window, the lodge cleaning crew were not about to open the door. When Tim lifted a trash can threatening to break the window, the crew decided to slip the key into the lock and open the door. "Call 911, there's been a terrible accident," he yelled.

This being a ski resort, the snow groomers were the first to the scene. Trained on rescue techniques, they knew how to handle the situation. Once the emergency team arrived, it took two snowmobiles and six rescue workers to get me out of the tree-infested embankment and down to the base of the mountain.

They say I was awake and communicating during the entire ordeal. But I can only remember a few vignettes of that night after my cry for help. The first was on a stretcher in the back of an ambulance. I held up my hands out from under a silver thermal blanket to look at them. My entire body was shivering. Apparently, my body temperature had dropped to the upper 80s—a situation I would later see as a benefit.

The next episode was in the emergency room. Someone was taking a stapler to my head. While ping-ponging through the trees, I picked up a gaping wound down the back of my head, just along the part of my pigtails. Evidently, staples were the tool of choice to close up the bleeding gash. I then went black.

Awakened again in the emergency room, I noticed I now had a Frankenstein-like helmet on my head and weights on my limbs. The pulling was unbelievably painful. The process of screwing the helmet onto my head reminded me of torture from the Middle Ages. Back to black.

My final emergency room memorable moment was when I awoke lying on my back in a white room. I had tubes everywhere and my eyes were wandering. To my right, I saw Tim. "I'm gonna get sick," I said. To ease the pain, the medical staff gave me morphine, a painkiller that does not agree with me. Tim looked around. "I'm gonna get sick," I reiterated.

Tim pressed the call button but no response. He stepped out to find a staff member. “She’s getting sick. Now!”

I don’t remember anything else from that evening. I’m told I was awake and communicating. I tend to think that my mind blocked out the rest and I don’t care to find out the other details. The damage was done.

Chapter 2: The Grief of Paralysis

The impact of a spinal cord injury is perplexing. Transitioning out of acute rehabilitation is a dichotomy. On one hand, you can't wait to get out of the hospital setting and get back to life as you know it. On the other hand, you are terrified to leave the comforts of the hospital care.

My cover was to celebrate my discharge from the hospital. "Crack open the champagne!" Home was the new frontier. The reality was as we drove back to our place in Manchester, I realized that life had changed, drastically. The front steps that I once hopped down for my morning runs had now turned into a major obstacle. That obstacle would make my current home feel like a prison.

Going home was surreal. The home that you thought would offer the comforts you were waiting to embrace again was not there. Home was filled with a space that was unfamiliar in my new state.

As we transitioned home, the accommodations for the wheelchair began to emerge. My family and Tim's were very supportive in this effort. Doors came off the hinges to make the passageways large enough for the wheelchair. Grab bars protruded from the walls. Transition ramps helped make the door thresholds passable. Then there was my closet filled with clothing I could no longer wear. Away went the heels and suits. But I kept my running sneakers.

This period of transition was a period of moving through the grieving process. It is not unlike grieving the loss of a loved one but in this case, I was grieving the lost use of my own body. In the field of psychology, there are defined stages of this process.

Elisabeth Kubler-Ross identified the five stages of grief: denial, anger, bargaining, depression, and acceptance. Although I insisted that I was different, I still went through those stages. What I didn't understand at the time is that everyone moves through them at a different pace. Some stages move quickly, others can linger. The key is to not get stuck in any one stage.

Denial

When the physician told me that I had an incomplete spinal cord injury and that I would be paralyzed and there is no cure, my first reaction was to deny the facts. I was different. Because I was incomplete, I could overcome this. It just bruised my spinal cord and bruises heal, right? The fact that I had an incomplete injury stuck in my head. I just had to work harder and I would be able to walk again. I had hope but I was denying the situation.

With this in mind, I would put more hours into rehabilitation than the next guy. I would get up at 5 am and start exercising right away. After dinner, I would go back to the gym and work again. My mom sent me a t-shirt that said "With perseverance and determination, anything can be achieved." I hung onto every word of that. Besides, before this accident, our life motto was "Work hard, play hard." Now, it was "Work hard, and work harder." Once outpatient physical therapy began, I would have transportation arranged to drive two hours each way just to get more physical therapy. In my mind, the rehabilitation process did not end at three months post-injury. I needed more therapy.

I focused on putting my life back together. Since working for a young technology company was a big part of that "normal" life, I wanted to get back to it. I denied that I was grieving and just needed to focus on working. This little accident was just a side hiccup. It will go away and I'll be back to normal before I know it. This was my state of mind until I moved back home. Then the next stage began.

Anger

Early on, I determined that I would *not* be a bitter person. I did not want to be that person walking around with a chip on her shoulder and angry at the world. But that stage of anger can creep into your life.

The bottom floor of the old colonial home where Tim and I lived was "suitable" for me to live in. Besides the 10 steps that went up to the front porch, the inside was navigable in a wheelchair. This house was built in the 1920s and the door passageways were wide. The home had pine wood flooring throughout, making it easy for wheeling the chair. The windows were low so I could look out at the world. The kitchen counter tops were high, but we moved everything to the lower cabinets. Besides, I was never alone and not ready to start cooking for myself.

The two bedrooms were big enough to maneuver the wheelchair. We had to rearrange some furniture in the bedroom that Tim and I shared but it worked. The other bedroom became my space. We set up a folding table with a mirror so I could do my hair and make-up. We took the extra futon, laid it out, and put it on stilts. This made a level transfer and an area for me to use for dressing.

Dressing was a challenge. Just trying to get a pair of pants on in a seated position was impossible. Jeans? Forget it. Zippers and buttons became daily obstacles. Velcro was my friend. The process of getting dressed was a one-hour ordeal. Add that into a morning routine of cathing, exercise, breakfast, and transfers, and it becomes a four-hour process just to get ready for the day. At the time, I had a caregiver come to the house but only in the evenings. I had to learn how to get myself dressed every day.

One morning I was getting ready to go to work. I was not driving yet and Tim would drive me and pick me up. I learned that I could shorten the dressing process by wearing a skirt and pulling it down over my head. I thought I was clever and could cut the time needed for getting dressed, but then I had to put on those shoes. Impossible. I couldn't get my leg up long enough to slip the shoe on the foot, but then the foot would swell and the shoe became a tight fit. After the fourth attempt to get that damn shoe on my foot, I took it and threw it as hard as I could across the room. The shoe hit the wall and bounced off the window, almost cracking it. The shoe was the problem, not me.

Anger came with my lack of independence or my new world of depending on others. The biggest obstacle was getting out of my house. Once Tim left for work for the day and the caregiver was not there, I was alone in the house. Those 10 steps from the front porch to the sidewalk was my obstacle. We rented a stair climber. It was an electronic mechanism that latched onto the wheelchair. Using tank-like treads, it would slowly walk me up and down those 10 steps. But I could not do this independently. Once alone in our house, I was imprisoned.

The imprisonment made me angry. Angry that I couldn't get out. Angry that the hospital dumped me into a home with no escape. Angry that I couldn't independently get dressed. Angry that people would talk to Tim and not me. Angry that there were not curb cuts at the end of the street. Angry that I couldn't drive the two cars that I owned. Angry that this incomplete injury wasn't healing fast enough. I didn't want to show that anger to the world and I released it in private. I was determined not to be the "bitter gimp." That anger turned into my bargaining chip.

Bargaining

My biggest bargaining target was the health insurance company. Here the power of negotiation and persistence paid off. I had health insurance through my employer, but it was a constant negotiation. The insurance company was trying to reduce costs and I was trying to get the best care. For traumatic cases such as a spinal cord injury, the insurance company assigned a case manager. Mine was named Judy.

Judy was a retired nurse. She was a woman of a medium build with dark hair and glasses. She was soft spoken and meticulous with her words. She would be the person to handle my case with the insurance company. She had her job to do, but the reality of the situation was that it was a cost control measure on the insurance side.

After returning home, our landlady paid us a visit to give some advice. Her son had Hodgkin's disease when he was young. She would stay at home from work to care for him and bargain with the insurance company to get the care he needed. She gave us many pieces of advice at the time. One of them was to appeal any denial from the insurance company and to get to know the state Insurance Commissioner.

I took that advice to heart and started bargaining for everything. At first, Judy was the target of negotiations. The insurance company wanted to stop paying for a personal care assistant. I had a PCA to help in the evenings with the shower and bowel routine. My bargaining tool: give me more occupational therapy sessions to learn the skills and then we can stop the PCA. That gave me more OT sessions to work on my hand dexterity. Judy would approve that. After about six months, Judy would "close" my case and move on to others with traumatic injuries. But I was not done bargaining.

The insurance company wanted to stop the rental of the stair climber. I bargained to keep it since the driver for my therapy had a bad back and Tim was at work. The insurance company wanted to stop therapy. I would work with my physical therapist to show that I was making small incremental improvements. The insurance company wanted to cover only four catheters per month. I would prove that I had infections and could not reuse "one-time use" catheters. My bargaining punching bag was the insurance company. In the end, it was the best way to use that emotional state to get the care I needed.

But not all bargaining worked to my advantage. Knowing that the home was a prison due to those 10 pesky steps, Tim and I started looking for more accessible places to rent. We found a new apartment complex on the other side of the river in Manchester, NH. The apartments were brand new and they had a one bedroom unit that was completely wheelchair accessible. The bathroom was big, doorways wide, entrance pathways easy. It was perfect. The problem: The unit was reserved for Section 8 housing. I made too much money to qualify for access to that unit. So, we negotiated.

"I'll give you cash for the unit now."

"No."

"I'll pay double the monthly rent."

"I'm sorry, we can't do that."

"I'll buy the unit from you."

"The unit is not for sale."

We were in a pickle. We did not have enough money at the time to buy property and build an accessible home. I made too much money to have access to accessible housing. Bargaining just didn't help.

My other area of bargaining was for a cure. There must be a cure for spinal cord injury. The hunt began. I started reading research journals, study results, and progress reports from research centers around the world. After countless hours of searching, there was no magic bullet out there.

But there were clinical trials. I started on a letter campaign to become a clinical trial participant. I'm motivated; I have a good support system; I show progress in therapy; I am young; I'm healthy; I'm bargaining to get myself into a cure trial. The responses slowly started to come back. It was like getting response letters from university entrance applications. "I'm sorry, we will not accept anyone less than one year post-injury." Period. That was the inclusion criteria and there was no way to negotiate that one. That bargaining chip was spent.

Depression

Depression was not a stage for me. I didn't hit depression and then get over it. For me depression crept in and out of my life. In the rehabilitation hospital, I would cry myself to sleep every night. And it continued when I went home. It was just harder because it became more difficult to hide from Tim. I would gauge my progression on how many times in a week I had to cry myself to sleep.

I would avoid the depression issue during the day. I would focus on work and therapy and staying busy so depression couldn't impact me. Regardless, it was the elephant in the room. At any moment, depression could rear its ugly head. I would cry if there was a paper jam in the printer. Break into tears if my meeting ran past my four-hour time mark to catheterize. Depression always seemed to be there, I would just push it down so it wouldn't surface. And maybe, just maybe, it would go away.

What I didn't realize at the time is that my family was going through the same difficult time dealing with my paralysis. Sometimes we forget that our "support system," friends and family members, are people too and they sometimes have to deal with depression themselves.

My feeling of helplessness continued. But it was not a constant. I would keep my dealings with depression very private. On the outside, I was strong and put up my armor. Inside I was crying like a baby. Over time, the cloud of depression went from overcast to broken to scattered cover. I never really got over the "hump" until about four years post-injury.

Stubborn as I am, I refused to use any pharmaceuticals. That would make me admit publically that I was struggling with depression. I did not go to a shrink, that would again mean admitting that I had an emotional issue. I never became suicidal. I just would let small things bother me. Even when I returned to work, I would take more bathroom breaks to go into the private stall and let out a few tears of relief. For a person like me who does not like to show public emotion, it was a difficult mask to wear.

Over time the sleeping giant subsided. Why or how it did, I simply don't know. Over time I came to terms with the accident, my situation, and how it impacted the people I love. Surely, the method I used to handle depression is not a healthy alternative. In the end, I went through depression, just not in a conventional way.

Acceptance

After the denial letters from research facilities stopped coming, I got the hint. There is no "cure" for spinal cord injury. *Okay.* That message got through my thick skull. *Now, what?*

In the acute rehabilitation process, rehabilitation staff members teach you about the plethora of secondary conditions after spinal cord injury. The battle moves from being "cured" and walking again to keeping the secondary conditions at bay. Statistically, it is not the spinal cord injury that kills people. It is the complications from secondary conditions that do kill people. For many years, the leading cause of death after spinal cord injury has been bladder infections and kidney failure.

Secondary conditions are complications from paralysis that adversely impact the body. The list of possible secondary conditions just seems endless: osteoporosis, contractures, muscle spasms, pressure sores, bladder infections, bowel compactions, obesity, pneumonia, and the list goes on. It can be overwhelming.

Unlike depression, my acceptance point was very distinct. "Okay, there is no cure for spinal cord injury. How do I keep myself healthy to combat the secondary conditions?" That's when I made the transition from rehabilitation to exercise. It is when I went from looking for that progress and getting frustrated when I realized that the exercise I was doing would keep me healthy.

My other motivating factor was this: When a cure for spinal cord injury *is* discovered, I want my body to be healthy and ready so I can be a candidate. If I sit around and let pressure sores occur and obesity take over and contractures lock my joints, I will never be a candidate for a spinal cord injury cure. That is the bottom line. That was my acceptance.

A Twitch of an Idea

The hunt transitioned from a search for the "cure" to a search for the best method to stay healthy. Earlier in my rehabilitation process, I was introduced to electrical stimulation. My first introduction came by way of my physical therapist, George, otherwise known as "Get your butt out of bed, George." He would come into my room at the rehabilitation hospital every morning and tell me that if I wanted to be in a manual wheelchair, I needed to exercise my arms to make that possible.

While I was still in the rehabilitation hospital, I wanted to exercise my paralyzed leg muscles. I had read about electrical stimulation so I asked George about it. He tested me with a small two-channel stimulator to see if I would respond to it. We put these little sticky pads on my front calf muscle and turned the system on. With the stimulation, my muscle contracted and my foot flexed up. That little twitch became my first movement via electrical stimulation. This could be useful, I thought.

That is what we did. At the time, I had very little movement in my hands. My wrists were getting stronger, but my fingers were so weak. I told the therapist that I wanted to be able to type again. So much of my work is on a computer that I couldn't do the two-finger tap. Using the two-channel stimulator, we placed the sticky pads on my forearm and began a regime to gain gross finger movements with electrical stimulation and coupled that with voluntary exercise. Eventually, I gained more finger function with the exception of my index fingers. It was a long process but it eventually worked.

So, here I am at this acceptance point in my life seeking a method to stay healthy. At the time functional electrical stimulation (FES) cycling was still new to rehabilitation hospitals. People did not have them in their homes. I did find an old FES cycle at a medical resale shop. It was in a warehouse filled with wheelchair parts and walkers. Tim and I went to look at it. They were selling it for a few thousand dollars and we would have to put a few more thousand into it to make it work and find a supplier of the sticky pads. It just was not feasible.

I finally found an FES cycle in a rehabilitation hospital in Massachusetts, about a three-hour drive south. I had to get on it. I was convinced that was what I needed.

To get access to the FES cycle, I needed a prescription from my doctor, transportation to the hospital, and approval from the insurance company. My insurance company eventually allotted a fixed amount of visits to use the FES cycle.

Voila! I was in business and able to attend a specific amount of FES cycling sessions. But those FES cycling sessions finally ran out and there were no functional outcome measures for the insurance company to approve more sessions. Decreased muscle spasms, improved circulation, less muscle atrophy were all considered "custodial" by the insurance company and not reimbursable outcomes. I then called about the FES cycle at the warehouse, but it was gone. Now, what? Appeal.

While working on about my third appeal against the insurance company to get more FES cycling sessions, I began researching medical publications about electrical stimulation. While hunting for justification for more electrical stimulation, I discovered the Cleveland FES Center. At the time, the institution included an FES Information Center. I called them and told them about my current mission.

After a few days, a large envelope arrived at my home with copies of research articles published about FES for spinal cord injury. Unlike the stimulation in FES cycles, which used electrodes placed on the surface of the skin, the Cleveland group was using surgically implanted electrodes to provide stimulation to paralyzed muscles. They also provided a listing of research programs currently being conducted at the FES Center. This was my introduction to the FES implanted Stand and Transfer program. I was on my way to becoming the first bionic woman.

Chapter 3: Clinical Trials and Tribulations

"I got in! I got in! I'm in!" Those were my first words after I read the news that I was accepted into the program. Wheeling out of my small home office into the living room, where Tim's Aunt AnnaLou was watching her evening episode of Jeopardy. I stopped at the threshold to the living room.

"I got in."

"Well, what did you get into Dear?"

"We're going to Cleveland. I was accepted into a research program."

"That's great, Dear."

I don't know if she fully understood what I was talking about or if I ever fully explained it. At that point, I was just elated to know there was some hope of moving on.

At the time, Tim was in Texas for one month of training with a new air cargo company. I had returned to work but was still not independent enough to stay at home by myself. While Tim was away at training, we flew Aunt AnnaLou from Florida to New Hampshire to stay with me and help me with the household duties that I was not able to perform. Plus, she was a fantastic chef and I enjoyed her evening meals and company.

The Application

Months prior I passed the one year post-injury threshold. It is an anniversary date that will live with you for the rest of your life. Some people celebrate, others cry; I tried my best not to get depressed but to reflect on the progress made from day one. While I was in my letter-writing campaign to research programs around the country, I wrote a letter to the principal investigator

(PI), Dr. Ron Triolo, at the Cleveland FES Center. The letter explained my physical state, nature of my injury, and reasons why I wanted to participate in a clinical research trial for spinal cord injury." *If not me, who? If not now, when?*

Accompanying the letter was a videotape. We made the tape to show evidence why I was a good candidate. In it was a demonstration of me getting up on KAFO (knee-ankle-foot orthosis) braces and using a swing-through gate to move around with a walker and the assistance of a caregiver. Also, on the tape were demonstrations of using a two-channel neuromuscular electric stimulator (NMES) on my lower limbs and how the muscles responded to the electrical stimulation.

On the first attempt, I received a rejection letter telling me they appreciated my contact but they had never implanted a woman and it was not appropriate for me to enter the program. Once I was past the initial disappointment, motivation kicked in. I sent a response letter making a case as to why women should be included in the program. "Twenty percent of spinal cord injuries are in women. If your program seeks to represent the SCI population, you will need to accept a woman into your program." Along with the case, I reiterated why I was the right candidate.

Several months after sending the second letter, a response came to me in the form of an invitation to come to Cleveland and be evaluated as a candidate into the program. They explained how there is a battery of tests to be done before acceptance into the program. Of the first order was to send my medical records to the Cleveland FES Center. With this instruction, I gathered the medical records from my injury date to present date including notes from the physical medicine and rehabilitation (PM&R) doctor and physical therapist. The large and bulging envelope was sent off to Cleveland.

Months passed again with a response of an invitation to visit Cleveland for testing. Tim and I took some time off work and booked flights to Cleveland. Thc trip was not only to the lab but we also paid a visit to my family, the majority of whom still lived in northeast Ohio. On our visit, my mom organized a gathering at her house with the family over the weekend. The weekday came and we had a tight schedule to keep.

The first visit was to the Louis Stokes Cleveland VA hospital. It is not in the best part of Cleveland with rundown crack houses across the street from the hospital. We parked and tried to find our way to the Motion Laboratory in the hospital. Down the elevator to the basement, the doors opened to hallways that were white with institutional linoleum floors and toothpaste-colored doorways. Proceeding through the maze we passed the dentist, eye care and the morgue before the hallway dead-ended at the Motion Laboratory door.

Upon entering the lab, we were greeted with members of the research team, including the physical therapist, principal investigator, and an engineer. After signing a stack of paperwork and liability releases, we then got to work. A discussion pursued about my medical history, my daily routine, and status of my health. The discussion also included the requirement to live in Cleveland if accepted into the program. At the time, research participants were not allowed to live outside of a short driving distance from Cleveland.

Finally, the real test began. The therapist sent me off to the restroom to change into shorts. Returning to the lab, they had a station set up on a therapy mat. I transferred onto the mat. The therapist explained the procedure while holding a probe covered in white cloth and a cup of water. They had me lie in various positions to get access to the targeted muscles. For instance, they placed a bolster under my knees and then placed the probe on my skin. Turning on the stimulation, my thigh muscles contracted, my knees straightened, and my foot was in the air. For each muscle group that they stimulated, a member of the research team recorded the response onto a hidden paper and clipboard. Along with every response, there was no indication of whether it was good or bad. They were neutral. At the conclusion of the tests, we were thanked for coming in. "The research team will discuss the results. Don't contact us, we will contact you." That was it. We got on the airplane and went back to New Hampshire with no hint as to what the result would be.

Months later, Tim was hired by an air cargo carrier and left for a month's worth of training. That's when the acceptance letter came. "I got in."

Accepted, now what?

Jennifer's Choice

You can't just be paralyzed for a year and expect the muscles to magically start working again like they did pre-injury. The research team gave me an exercise schedule. The exercise was spearheaded by a two-channel neuromuscular electrical stimulator. It is a small unit to which two wires are connected with surface electrodes attached to them. Over a period of time, I was to use the NMES system to exercise each muscle group that was targeted for a surgical implant. I had instructions for each day and had to record what exercises were actually performed.

Then came the arrangements. After talking with Tim and calling family members, we had to figure how we could make this happen. But there were a few things Tim and I needed to discuss before turning our lives upside down and moving to Cleveland.

On the top of the topic list was children. We weren't married at the time but both knew in the back of our minds that one day we would join the category of "married" at some point in the future. But what about children? In order to be a participant in this research project, I had to agree (and legally sign) that I would not become pregnant. If I did, the system would need to be explanted. More importantly, there was no known impact of electrical stimulation to an unborn child. The question loomed; do we want children?

That little check box on the legal documents to enter a clinical trial sparked a life journey conversation between Tim and me. We discussed pregnancy as a quadriplegic; the fact that we may not be ready now but what about the future; and alternative options like adoption, surrogate mother, artificial insemination. Aside from the other logistical things we needed to attend to, the childbirth conversation was concentrated into several hours. It wasn't one of those looming topics that you discuss, sleep on it, and then return to at a later date. No, this was one that we needed to hash out, make a decision, and move on. It didn't need to involve anyone else. This was simply a decision between Tim and me.

The verdict: we chose not to have children. If we changed our minds in the future, then we would either adopt or find a surrogate mother. (Later my sister stepped up and volunteered to be one if we chose to go that route). Done. Time to move on to logistics.

At the time, in order to join this research project, the participant had to live within a defined radius of the research center. That meant if I wanted these implants, then we would need to pick up our lives in New Hampshire and move to Northeast Ohio. People move all the time due to work but this was different. We were moving our lives for the hope that some unknown technology could improve my life as a quadriplegic.

It wasn't proven. It wasn't a guarantee. It wasn't like I had a desk and a job waiting for me at the other end. The details of our lives had to be arranged within the complexity of living with a disability.

We thought finding housing when I moved from the hospital to home life was difficult—now we had to find a place to live in Northeast Ohio that was wheelchair-accessible. It's not like you can call a condominium complex sales office and say, "Hi, I'm looking for a wheelchair-accessible condo. Do you have any available?" Using that approach would only yield an answer like, "No, but there is a nursing home down the street."

I am still amazed at how far behind we are as a society when it comes to integrating people with disabilities into our homes. Eventually, we found a new apartment complex in Parma Heights, a suburb of Cleveland. It was not "wheelchair accessible" but it was adaptable for me to live independently for the required 18 month term. It was a 15-minute drive to the hospital where I would spend countless hours. It was 15 minutes to the airport for an easy commute for Tim. Plus, it bordered the Metro Park system so I had access to biking trails. It was not in the best part of town but not in the worst. It was a temporary move and we made it work for us.

The other logistics seemed to fall in place. It took some work but we made it happen. At the time, Tim was working for an air freight company and I was back to work at PC Connection. For Tim, we simply applied to change his based airport from Boston to Cleveland. It took some paperwork. For me, it took some compromising.

Since I was working from home and the company already had a satellite office in southern Ohio, it was possible to still work for the company as an employee. At this time, I already was working from home on a part-time basis; mostly when the snow was high and the plows were delayed getting to my street. We finally came up with an agreement between PC Connection and me that worked for both of us. It was an unusual situation and I am forever grateful to an organization that looked outside the norm to help an employee. I would work from home full-time and travel back to the New Hampshire office on a set schedule.

Scheduling was a project of commitment. Not just for work but for the research project. After being accepted into the program, they gave me a flow diagram depicting the various stages from surgery through discharge, along with the time commitment for each stage. That gave me a clear view of the time needed to get this technology. That's when it really penetrated my skull that this was a big commitment. Truth be told, it only scratched the surface. The rehabilitation phase would be riddled with extra experiments, additional testing, and demonstrations, but that was not neatly drawn on this initial diagram. Time would end up being the biggest asset and the biggest contribution to the research project. At the time, I had no idea how valuable that time really was.

The value was not just the giving of time. We also had a big financial commitment. Tim and I moved our lives to Cleveland. The move was out of our pockets; no one paid for that. Expenses like transportation to and from the hospital, housing, parking fees, airline tickets, and toll fees were all out of our pockets. There was no expense report to submit for reimbursement. We paid the expenses from our own pockets and took a medical deduction on tax day. I've never added up all the receipts from the time I joined the project until discharge. I probably don't want to know. What I did know is that taking the plunge to get this technology (that may or may not work) was a financial commitment from us.

Countdown to Surgery

While all of these logistical points were being hashed out, the research team was still trying to come up with a surgery date. At the time, I still did not know when we would pick up our lives and move. It was almost like waiting for a military deployment date. Not knowing your future schedule can be very frustrating, particularly when working in a world where schedules are set months in advance.

Finally, the date was set: November 11, 1999. That was it. I would be implanted on Veterans Day. Everything started to fall into place from there. Tim rented a U-Haul truck. We recruited some friends. When moving day came, we loaded up the truck and my vehicle and headed west to Ohio. We said our goodbyes to friends. We took one last look at the empty space in the bottom of the old Colonial home. It was the place where I went through so many emotions in the transition from upright to seated life. It was time to let go and move on.

It was the fall; the trees were in full brilliant colors as Mother Earth transitioned from summer to winter. The trip from New England to the Great Lakes marked a rite of passage in our lives. Tim and I drove through to arrive in Cleveland on October 25. It was a 1 ½ weeks before the surgery date.

One benefit of the research project being in Cleveland was that I was close to my immediate family. That support system kicked into action to help Tim and I settle into the new living quarters. The paperwork stated that the bottom floor apartment was "move-in" ready but for a wheelchair user, the work had only just begun.

For instance, the carpeting was plush, which made it very difficult to propel my wheelchair. We did not have the option of taking it out or even buying different carpeting. So, we laid peg board down on common routes around the apartment. The board was dull brown, but it did the job of make moving around the living space possible for me. Later, my sister would paint rugs and various designs on the board in an attempt to make it appear more pleasant. Eventually, we figured out a routine for me to live relatively independently in this new area.

Getting Implanted

With all the commotion of moving and settling in, the surgery date approached without much fanfare or thought on my part. I was so pre-occupied with trying to pull our new life together that I never saw the surgery date approaching with any anticipation. Sure there was pre-op testing but it was just another doctor visit to me.

A few days prior to the surgical implant, I was brought in to meet some members of the research team. The appointment was technically not for that but more for paperwork. A stack of legal documents were placed in front of me. There were the liability releases, research participant agreements, and basic commitments that I would need to acknowledge and sign in order to give me access to this new technology. It was not just putting my initials on page 6, 15, 37, and 79. Nope, each and every word had to be read to me, acknowledged, and then each page initialed by me. So, the physical therapist, Carol, sat next to me and dictated the entire stack of legal documents to me. She made sure I understood *all* of my commitments to the program. It took hours. It was not only laborious for me, but for Carol, who really had the tough job. For me, it spelled out every detail and consequence. And there were no cliff notes or short cuts.

The date just came. It was a Thursday. Tim was on the second half of his two-week road tour. I was making final arrangements to be “on vacation” for a week. The night before the implant, I arrived at MetroHealth Medical Center and navigated through the hospital maze to find the CRC (Clinical Research Center). It was a small section of the hospital dedicated to human clinical research. The outside looked intimidating. There was a front office and next to it double doors much like those you would see marking the entrance to an emergency room. The waiting room was dark with typical hospital waiting room chairs and a small area dedicated to administration.

There was a woman at the desk with a welcoming smile. When I entered, she looked up and said, "You must be Jennifer. We've been expecting you." After answering a battery of questions, she led me through a door to the research ward. It was a short hallway with three inpatient rooms on one side and a supply room door on the other. She escorted me to the middle room. "Here you go."

The room was a typical hospital room decorated in true 1980s flare with mauve pinks, dull blues, and teal green. There was a window that overlooked the top of some old building. It would be a window I would look at often in the days to come.

"We call this the Reeve room. Christopher Reeve stayed here. Make yourself at home and the therapist will be in to see you." The ward was quiet, unlike a typical hospital. There was no one there. Empty. You could not even hear the beeps, pages, and noises from the rest of the hospital. Occasionally, you would hear a helicopter and then smell the fumes, but that was about it.

The therapist came in to check on me. She went over some paperwork and made sure I had what I needed for the evening. I was told no eating or drinking. She told me to get a good night's sleep and the team would be in the next morning. And then she left. I changed into the hospital gown and asked the nurse to help me transfer into bed. Then I went to sleep. I had no idea what I was getting into but somehow I was comfortable with the decision. I closed my eyes to get a few hours of sleep.

Six am came quickly. The lights came on with the words, "Your time is here." Two interns walked into the room with a transport bed. Before I could get ready and awake, they transferred me into the transport bed and off I went. "Are you comfortable, dear?" I shook my head yes. "Good, because you're going for a ride." Through the double doors to the CRC we went, down an elevator, weaving through the maze of hallways but all I could see was the white foamboard ceiling and occasional florescent lights. I had no idea where I was but it looked like the deep bowels of a hospital. At that point, it registered in my brain that I was now going into surgery.

The rendezvous ended at the pre-op room. Behind a shield of glass, there was a big room with curtains separating the long wall into waiting stalls. In each stall, there were people in beds awaiting their turn for the operating room. Some were sleeping, others had the look of anxiety and some had family hovered around. They placed me is a waiting stall at the end of the row with a curtain making one side and a white wall making the other.

Visitors starting coming into my stall. Each came for a short time and went back out quickly. First a nurse, holding paperwork, checking my wristband and asking me questions. Then the PI asking me how I was doing. The IV nurse came in with needles and fluids. Then a person in a white coat checked my vitals. Then the therapist came in and left. The PI came in again and then back out. I felt like my stall was a revolving door. Questions were asked with no time to think but instinct blurted out an answer. Perhaps that's what they wanted.

At one point, I peeked past the curtain to see a crowd of people peering through the glass wall. Each was on a visitor list. The visitor list was not for the various people down pre-op row awaiting surgery. Oh, no. That long list of visitors was for me—people approved to observe the implantation surgery. There was definitely an audience for this ordeal. Finally, the PT came back in with my mom.

"Everything is fine." The PT assured me. "I will keep your mom informed throughout the surgery."

"I'll call Tim and let him know too," my mom chimed in. Tim was on the road as part of his tour of piloting duty. We planned for him to be on the road while I was in the hospital and then home for two weeks once I was discharged. There was no reason for him to be home while I was laid-up in a hospital. All he would do is pace the halls. Besides, after my initial injury, he had had enough of being in hospitals.

At that point, I was already starting to feel the effects of the pre-op anesthesia they had given me through the IV. "That's fine." I said. With that, I was told to count backwards from 100... and I was out.

Seven and a half hours later, I was in the recovery room with the most awful hangover. I thought I had some pretty bad ones in college after an evening of drinking tequila. But this was the mother of all hangovers. My vitals must have checked out and my body stabilized. I don't remember much of the recovery room and was brought back to the Reeve room.

For two days, I tried to sleep off the hangover. The room was kept dark. Periodically, a nurse would come in to check on me and take my vitals, but I don't remember. There were occasional visitors from the research team, medical staff or my family, but I don't remember them either. I was in pain. Not from the surgery or the multitude of incisions but from the anesthesia. It wasn't until the second day when I puked my guts out that I began to feel better.

On Sunday, I was feeling better and conscious of the world around me. That evening, Tim appeared with his pilot uniform on and his designated rollie bag.

"Hi. How are you?"

"Okay. How did you get here?"

"RTA bus. Taking the bus in downtown Cleveland is a scary thing." With that, he put down his bag and began to tell me about how he got from Cleveland Hopkins airport to MetroHealth Medical Center via the bus system. He told me about how he got lost, how he finally figured out where he was, and how he may have been exposed to infectious diseases like TB. While he was talking, my eyes must have been nodding off.

He said. "Okay, enough of that. I'll let you sleep. Give me a few days to get settled and I'll be back in."

"Okay. Thanks for coming in. Love you." He gave me a kiss and walked back out the door.

The First Stand

It was Monday; four days after the surgery. At this point, I was eating hospital food, drinking water, and getting up with the help of the physical therapists. On this day, there was a visit from several members of the research team. They came in with clipboards and electrical equipment. It was easy to pick out the engineers in the group; they had the electrical equipment in hand. They all circled around the hospital bed, while the PI stood back against the wall. He was observant but let his team do their work.

"Today, we would like to test your system," announced one of the engineers. "We are going to run a few tests, if it is okay with you."

I thought, *What else do I have to do?* "Sure, go ahead," is what actually came out of my mouth. With that approval, they started testing. At the time, I really did not know what they were testing or what data they were collecting, but in the end it all looked official. There were a lot of "hmms" and "oohs" sprinkled in with technical jargon, but nothing that made sense to me.

Finally, the physical therapist said that they wanted to test my quadriceps muscles. There was a reason they wanted me to do the pre-surgical exercises. As it turns out, during the surgery before implanting an electrode, the team turns on the electrode, which contracts the muscle. The electrode is not sutured to the muscle until the therapist has given final approval. Now, they wanted to see if they could get the same muscle contraction as the one they had during the surgery. The PT placed a bolster under my knees while the engineer held a coil over the left side of my abdomen just over the area that held the implanted receiver.

"Are you ready?" the PT asked while she held my ankle and braced my knee.

"Um, sure." With the click of a button, my left leg kicked out straight into the air. My eyes widened. This was the first time I had seen my leg move after the injury. It moved without someone else doing the act. It moved without having a mechanical brace attached to it. It was just me looking at my leg with my thigh muscle fully contracted. It was the most beautiful thing I had seen in a year and a half—my leg moving under my own muscle power. Yes, there was a mechanical implanted thing in me making it happen, but at the time it didn't matter. What mattered was that I was looking at my own muscle contracting and my own leg kicked out, defying gravity.

With a second click of the button, the system turned off and my leg was back on the bolster, paralyzed as before. "Would you do that again?" I asked. I just had to see it another time. I had to know that it was real. They did do it again, and again, and again. After several tests with both legs, they got the information they needed and called it a wrap.

After seven days in the hospital, they released me to go home for the remainder of the recovery period. For eight weeks, I was on restricted activity. Restricted activity consisted of two transfers per day (into the wheelchair from bed was considered one transfer), no bending of more than 45 degrees from front or either side and no heavy lifting.

This is when the support system becomes so important. Without the overwhelming support from my family and friends, the process would be so different and difficult. For the first two weeks, Tim was home and helped me with my restrictions. For the second two weeks, Tim's mom, Betty, flew in from New York to help me. That gave me a chance to spend time with my future mother-in-law. For the third two weeks, Tim was back home. For the final two weeks, I got by on my own with occasional visits from my mother, father, and sister. During this recovery time, I was back to working from home. The time seems to pass quickly since I was preoccupied with my work.

Once the eight weeks passed, I returned to MetroHealth Medical Center for a checkup. That checkup consisted of some long testing sessions, some medical testing of vitals, and (the most important) my exercise plan. In order to build up muscle tissue, the therapist game me a progressive exercise routine using the newly implanted electrodes. The exercise routine consisted of leg lifts with progressive weights, glut and back exercises, and endurance exercises. Each was designed to build various muscle tissue prior to a first stand with the system.

That was the goal. Build up to be able to stand with the implanted system. Standing was my motivation to do the exercises on a daily basis. It was the carrot the therapist hung to get me to do the exercises. Standing was the goal. For the next six weeks, I would be performing the exercises to build up to the initial stand date. Unlike the pre-surgery exercises, these had a purpose. Sure, the pre-surgery exercises had the purpose of preparing the muscles for surgery. But now, I had a taste of what this new system could do. I saw my leg kick out. Now, I had a true goal of exercise: get the muscles strong enough to stand. That was something tangible that I could envision.

It was the middle of February and the research team gathered around the lab. Plus, my mom, father, and Tim joined me on this laboratory visit for my first stand date. As with anything, we don't just flip the switch and everything works. No, we spent the first half of the day running tests to tweak the system. After several hours on the therapy mat and test after test after test, we finally had the parameters dialed in to the desired settings and the possibilities looked good. The stand was a go.

The team gathered around; the research team along with members of my support team. Even the surgeon came in to see the results. He was the first to notice. "You have a new addition to your finger." Over the New Year's holiday, Tim proposed to me and we agreed to get married at some future date. "No date is set yet."

The therapist and I went to the parallel bars while the engineers stood by. Of course, the cameras and video cameras were set to capture the moment. The therapist reviewed the procedure and how we would go about doing a stand with the system. She would control the buttons. I needed to hold on to the parallel bars and let the system do the work. "Easy for you to say," I thought. Everyone was in position.

Beep.

A few seconds later.

Liftoff!

I was up. I looked down at my feet then looked over at my family. With a big smile I said, "Look, Ma, no braces." That was the first thing I noticed. I was standing upright on my own two legs, no standing frame, no braces, just my legs. Wow. After a few seconds, I sat back down. Gleeful and filled with joy, I asked to do it again. The therapist agreed but warned that we don't want to fatigue the muscles. I didn't care about fatigue. I just wanted to experience that again.

Life as a Swinger

That night, I went home with this deep sense of satisfaction. After all the letter-writing, arrangement making, people-coordinating, and simply picking up our lives, the goal was reached. I was able to stand.

Now, I wanted more.

Over time, I did get more. Eventually, I moved from standing in the parallel bars to standing with a walker. Standing eventually moved to being able to transfer (get in and out of the wheelchair) from one place to another. Gradually, transferring progressed to moving around short distances with a swing-through gait. Holding the walker with both arms, I would "swing" both legs simultaneously, thus propelling my body forward. I wasn't actually taking steps, per se, but to me it was still one giant leap for (wo)mankind.

After gaining their trust and my own, I was now standing and moving around independently. With that came a release to use the system at home and in the environment. I was released. Now came the exploration of how to use this new system in everyday life.

As I became more comfortable with the system, I began to use it more. At home, it was useful for reaching things that were out of reach. But I tried more "tricks" as Tim would start to call them. Home tasks like emptying the dishwasher or cleaning; it was useful.

But out of the home is where the rubber met the road. Ever stand at the seventh inning stretch at a baseball game? I could now. How about a standing ovation at a concert? Done. In the real world, there are many instances where the wheelchair just doesn't cut it and the standing system becomes a valuable asset.

I was on the hunt for milestones like that. The biggest onc of them all was on October 6, 2001—our wedding day.

I didn't use the system to just stand at the altar. Oh no. It

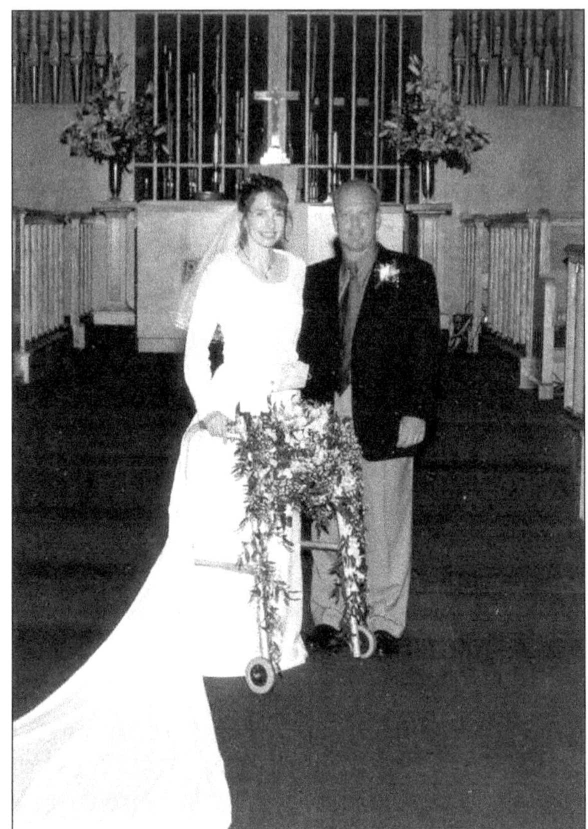

I used the system to walk down the aisle at my wedding.

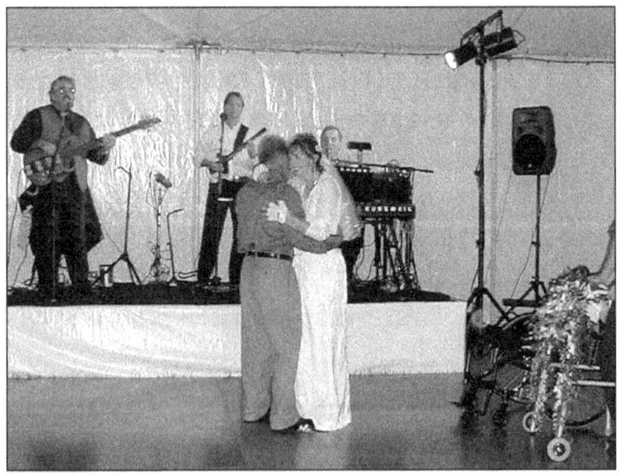

Our first dance

was much more than that. There was no wheelchair in our entire wedding ceremony. I used the system to walk down the aisle with my Dad. I used the system to stand at the altar and exchange vows.

My walker was decorated like a bride's bouquet. For the ceremony, I was not a wheelchair user. Because of this system, I left my wheelchair behind, left my paralysis behind, and enjoyed our wedding like any other bride.

Unexpectedly and completely not planned nor rehearsed, Tim and I decided to have out first dance using the system. It was actually Tim's idea and he had to convince me it was right. "Come on," he said. "I'll have you."

Out in front of our family and friends, I stood from the wheelchair in the middle of the dance floor. I put my arms around Tim and a friend of ours took the walker away. It was just us; no metal, no wheels, just us. I don't even think I heard the music. I was too focused on us. With that, the system gave us a moment we will never forget.

System Components

The stand and transfer system consists of both implanted and external components. It has eight channels—one for each electrode. The implanted components include electrodes—in and on the surface of the muscle—implanted deep into the muscle tissue. They were carefully placed by the research team mainly where the peripheral nerve innervates the muscle. The electrodes are placed in the quadriceps, hamstrings, gluteus maximus, and the lower back. It is bilateral—there is a set for the right side of the body and the left.

From each electrode extends a small, stretchy wire. These wires tunnel through the fatty tissue up to the left hip area where they connect to an implanted receiver. This receiver is sutured to the tissue under the skin and connects to all the electrodes, like a hub.

The external components consist of a coil taped to the skin over the receiver and an external control unit that is about the size of a small cable modem. The external control unit is the

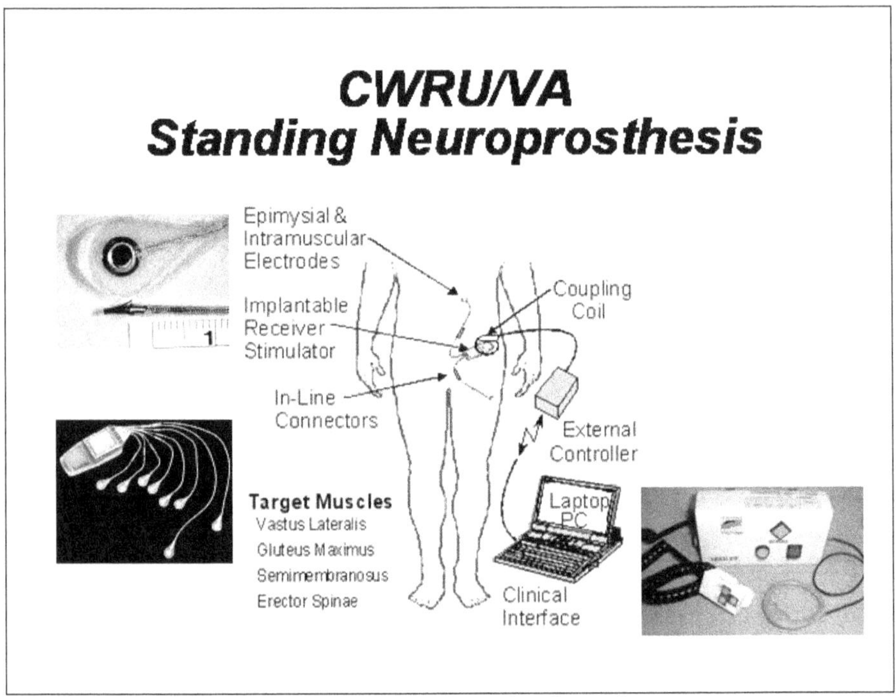

Components of the implanted eight-channel stand and transfer system

"brain" of the system. It holds the circuit boards and the power source for the system. When activated, the control unit sends messages via high-frequency radio signals through the coil to the implanted receiver. The receiver decodes the message and sends signals to the electrodes, activating the electrodes and stimulating the muscles to fulfill the given function.

The system has several functions from which the user may choose. Of course, it allows for activation of muscles to stand with a walker. It has other useful functions, as well. Leg lift exercises build the quads. An **Extends All** function activates all the muscles on for 10 seconds and then off for 10 seconds for a patterned duration of one hour. This builds endurance fibers in the muscles and helps reduce spasticity.

Revisions

After a while, I was discharged from the program and was now free to use the system. The research team continued to monitor my use and replace any broken equipment, but the weekly therapy visits were done.

Over the years of using the system, it became integrated into my daily life. Taping electrical coils to my skin is part of my daily routine. In January, 2003, I started to notice that my standing times were decreasing and I was not as stable as I once was. With this concern, I contacted the FES Center.

After paying a visit to the laboratory, we discovered that I was still standing but not with the original eight electrodes. At that time, I was down to five electrodes. There were two that were inoperative and one that became very weak. After several days of testing and hours of discussions the research team and I decided to conduct a revision surgery to get the system back to full capacity.

I'm not sure how they did it, but revisions are not part of a research grant. In fact, maintenance is not part of research. With the many medical devices being tested today, people volunteer their bodies and use the devices as part of a research project. Regardless of what functional gain the participants have or what condition it addresses, when the research is over, that's it. No maintenance funding exists. System revisions are not part of protocol. As a participant, you're out of luck.

But somehow working within this uniquely American funding structure, the FES Center found a way to provide me with a revision surgery and get me back to capacity.

Again around a holiday, the revision surgery was scheduled for Columbus Day, October 2003. This time, it was a little different. The surgery was only to replace three electrodes so it couldn't possibly be that bad. I felt very casual about it. I knew exactly what I was getting into. That may have been the problem.

Just before departing for the hospital for the surgery, I felt a wave of anxiety. With that wave, I went into the bathroom and proceeded to dry-heave into the toilet. When I was done, I washed my mouth out, fixed my hair, and proceeded to the hospital like nothing happened.

The same post-surgery procedures ensued. The procedure took seven hours of operating room time. But this time, they had a hard time getting me to wake up. As any baseball fan knows, October is playoff season. It's the run up to the World Series. I had seven days in the hospital to watch the Florida Marlins against the Chicago Cubs and more importantly, the New York Yankees against my beloved Boston Red Sox. Post surgery, they could not get me to snap out of my anesthesia coma.

The PI knew exactly what to do. He bent down to my ear and said, "Jen, the Red Sox just beat the Yankees." Instantly, I was awake, "No way!" It did the trick.

As the weeks progressed, I would visit the lab for testing and eventually got back on my feet. The revision worked and I was functionally standing again—as good as new. Once again, I was released from the program to test the system in the outside world and push it to the limits. I had another great seven years of using the system, integrating it into my daily life, and reaping the rewards of discoveries of medical research.

Chapter 4: The Second Generation

On March 13, 1998, I sustained a spinal cord injury from a snowboarding accident. This accident left me a quadriplegic. To say the least, it was life changing.

For 11 of the years post-injury, I used a stand and transfer neural prosthesis. I was the first woman to receive such a system. It consists of implanted electrodes that stimulate my paralyzed muscles and an external control device.

Using this device on a daily basis gave me the ability to keep my paralyzed muscles healthy while combating medical complications common among people living with spinal cord injuries, such as pressure sores, spasticity, and muscle atrophy. The neuroprosthetic system also offered me alternatives to my wheelchair by enabling me to move around short distances with a walker.

I've had some unique experiences with this system that many medical experts might have considered impossible upon my initial diagnosis: standing for the seventh inning stretch at a baseball game, standing to hug a loved one, or walking down the aisle at our wedding. I integrated this technology into my daily life and grew accustomed to its benefits.

But in 2010, it became time for an upgrade. Upgrading an implanted neurological device is not as simple as upgrading your cell phone or computer. It would require hours of exercise, therapy, and a lengthy surgical procedure.

On August 30, 2010, a talented team at the Cleveland FES Center scheduled to implant the upgraded system. The surgery was expected to take seven hours with six weeks of recovery followed by rehabilitation and testing. The entire process would take about a year, beginning in July 2010, when I started a four-hour daily exercise protocol. During this time, I kept a journal chronicling the experience and posted the entries to an on-line blog. Much of what follows in this book was adapted from that blog.

Why the Upgrade?

A member of the research team asked me, "Why do you want to go through with this?" The answer is not as easy as "Because I want to." There are several reasons, some more practical than others.

The first-generation system had eight channels. Before the upgrade, one electrode was turned off, the right hamstring. There was another electrode functioning at an extremely low level, the right glut. In essence, in 2010 I was standing on six electrodes rather than eight. It impacted my standing endurance; reducing the maximum stand time from 45 minutes to just 20 minutes. An average transfer took less than 30 seconds, so it was still "functional," but I had become accustomed to using it for longer periods of time.

Since I was lopsided on electrodes, standing put strain on my right quadriceps and my right knee tended to bend unexpectedly while standing. This required me to keep both hands on the walker at all times and I no longer felt safe using single-handed standing—to get objects out of reach for instance. For this reason, the system was not completely functioning to its original potential.

Age of the system was another consideration. Can you imagine using a cell phone that is 11 years old? I know many iPhone users who can't handle one that is more than 18 months old. The implanted system was still safe and "useable" but I had this inherent desire for the latest available technology if it could offer a better alternative. Marketers of consumer electronics are all too familiar with this human behavior. In this case, it is a little different. How long could I continue to use the first-generation system? If it had failed, would I go back to the long leg plastic braces I was using before the original implant? I had become almost addicted to the system; it was integrated into my daily life.

With spinal cord injury, many people focus on just the paralysis, the non-use of a limb, but there is more to it. As you learn in rehab, there is also a daily management of or daily fight against secondary health complications like osteoporosis, pressure sores, joint contractures, urinary infections, spasticity, and poor blood circulation to name a few. Some of these can be silent killers or major life disruptions. Over the years, I've lost friends to some of these complications. There are alternative means to manage these secondary conditions and many people living with spinal cord injury do so. The point is that I manage them using the implanted system. Without it, I would need to totally change how I ward off those common secondary complications.

Finally, what was my alternative? I had made a choice many years ago to become actively involved with the advancement of science for spinal cord injury. I don't have the mental capacity to be a scientific researcher or the training, for that matter.

When I was a student working on my MBA, I attended a talk given by the former CEO of Revlon. She highlighted a theme that stuck with me: "If not me, who? If not now, when?" That guided me in becoming a clinical trial participant and knowing the many risks and responsibilities that accompany that role.

While deciding whether to upgrade to the next generation system, I did another search of the current alternatives for people with chronic spinal cord injury? Yes, people have paid thousands of dollars to go to countries such as China, India, and Mexico to have stem cells implanted. Most recently, the FDA cleared Geron to continue a human clinical trial in the U.S. I was too chicken to do that and I did not completely understand the mechanisms and potential results. There have been some promising developments in gene therapies, but that line of research is still in the early stages and did not apply to humans yet. New rehabilitation techniques have emerged; but my injury is too chronic and complete for it to apply to my case. To me, upgrading my stand and transfer system was the best alternative at the time.

Plus, as a childhood viewer of Lindsey Wagner in 'The Bionic Woman," it was pretty cool to experience it firsthand.

Expanding from 8 to 24

Let's go over the plans for the new system and account for the 24 channels.

First, we kept the original eight-channel system. It consists of eight electrodes along with a receiver called an IRS-8. The IRS-8 receiver is implanted in the front left lower abdominal area. We kept the old system for several reasons:

- It still works, so why toss it out?
- If we go in to change it, we run the risk of damaging one or more components.
- My peace of mind. If all else fails, we can go back to the old system.

So that's the first eight of the 24 channels.

For the next 16 channels, we implanted an additional receiver, the IST-16, in the right front lower abdominal area. Yes, the name says it all; the device receives power and control information from outside the body and generates 16 channels of stimulation. The newly implanted electrodes connect to the IST-16 (I can hear the marketers out there cringing).

The new system consists of two types of electrodes: cuff and intramuscular. Just as it sounds, the cuff electrode is the shape of a spiral. In this spiral, there are four individual electrical contacts. The cuff electrodes are implanted on the left and right sides to control the group of muscles that comprise the quadriceps. Yes, I already had electrodes implanted in the quadriceps but those are intramuscular. By implanting the cuff electrode we expected to selectively stimulate

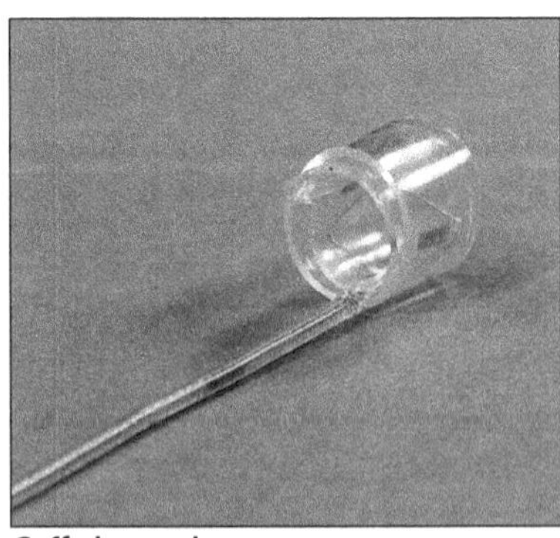

Cuff electrode

muscles within the quadriceps and potentially increase strength and endurance. Each cuff has four channels—one for each point of contact—making a total of eight channels. On our count up to 24, we now have 16.

The remaining eight channels were allocated to single channel intramuscular electrodes. They would be implanted as follows:

- Left and right posterior portion of adductor magnus (the inner thigh)
- Left and right gluteus medius
- Left and right quadratus lumborum (lower back muscles)
- Right hamstring
- Right gluteus maximus

Final calculations: eight channels of intramuscular electrodes, eight channels in the two cuff electrodes and the original eight-channel system. It all adds up to a 24-channel system. This would be the starting point for the surgical team since the plan may need to be adjusted in the operating room to get the best result.

Surgery was now less than four weeks away!

Chapter 5: Getting a Baseline

Testing was a big part of this entire research project. A significant factor to move forward was the baseline testing during a visit to Cleveland in March 2010. The results from this testing were pivotal because it determined if I would be a candidate for the new system. At the time, I was 12 years post injury and I couldn't be guaranteed candidacy.

During this session, members of the research team and I tested several factors, including the current system, the potential areas of implantation with surface stimulation, and factors relating to trunk control.

Testing of the current system was performed to understand the thresholds of each muscle currently implanted with an electrode. We tested the strength of the muscles on the Ashworth scale, which is commonly used by physical therapists to grade muscles on a scale of 0 to 5. The grade is assigned after the electrode is turned on. The thresholds are determined by testing the lowest setting when a muscle contraction begins and the highest setting that can be tolerated by the user (me). All of this data is recorded to use as a baseline, which is necessary to determine if there is improvement or not with the new system. For example, the first-generation system has two intramuscular electrodes implanted in the lower back area whereas the new system would add intramuscular electrodes in the same general area. The idea is to see if there is improved trunk control with the additional electrodes.

To test the potential area of implantation, the research therapist used a stimulation probe to find the key points on the surface of the skin to gain the desired muscle contraction. The gluteus medius, for example, will push the leg out in a scissor motion when it is contracted. Using a probe, the therapist located and marked the optimum spot for a muscle contraction on the surface of my skin and then placed a surface electrode on that specific spot.

Once each area was tested and located individually, we then combined them to create a standing system. One of the engineers did some magic to program an external control unit to direct the surface electrodes and the implanted electrodes. Using this "prototype" system, I was able to stand and get a sneak peak of what the new system would do and if my body would respond to it.

Finally, testing trunk control was an important potential functional gain. Trunk control—or the lack of it—is difficult to describe to able-bodied folks. It's relatively easy for a non-paralyzed person to understand the perspective of a wheelchair user—just let them use a wheelchair for a day. But simulating lack of trunk control is more difficult. For those who participate in Yoga, Pilates, or activities of that nature, you understand the importance of "core muscles" in your torso. For some people with spinal cord injuries, those core muscles are not functioning voluntarily. With my implanted system, there is a means to restore function in those core muscles. To gather a baseline prior to surgery, we did some testing on the venerable dynamometer machine, with which I would become quite familiar in the ensuing months. Using the dynamometer, we did several tests to gather data on the current function, strength, and endurance of my trunk muscles.

Preparation for Surgery

They say good preparation leads to successful outcomes and quicker recovery. Sometimes we have the premonition that just having a surgical procedure will fix a health issue. That knee replacement will help a person walk again or stomach bypass surgery will fix weight problems. In reality, it is not the surgical procedure alone. A component of a successful outcome is truly dictated by the attitude, behavior, and participation for the recipient. Surgery is one component that can help improve health, but it is not a panacea. Weight management includes exercise, food intake, and lifestyle changes. The surgery to upgrade my implanted neuroprosthesis was no different. It would not be the answer to all issues related to spinal cord injury, but the expected outcome would help my daily function and long-term health.

Since mid-July of 2010, I had been "laying low." I reduced my activities to create time to prepare for the surgery on August 30. Preparation not only included mental functions, arranging to be on "limited activity" post surgery, but also exercise. The research protocol called for exercise of the paralyzed muscles that were targeted to be implanted at least 30 days prior to surgery. So beginning on July 29, I had to comply with a 4¾ hour daily exercise protocol. I actually started in mid-July. Starting early helped with the daily adjustment, especially since in the first few weeks, I cheated and skipped several exercises. Those extra few weeks of exercise helped me adjust my daily living activities to make sure I did not miss any of the exercises for the day.

So, what am I exercising for that many hours? First targets are the muscles that already have electrodes implanted in them. Here are the exercises I performed using the first-generation implanted system:

- Leg lifts to exercise the quadriceps: 30 minutes
- Hips and backs exercises for the gluteus maximus, hamstrings, and back muscles: 30 minutes
- Standing: 30 minutes
- Extends All (which builds endurance fibers in all implanted muscles): 60 minutes

That adds up to 2½ hours per day.

In addition, the research team issued me a two-channel neuromuscular stimulator. The device delivers electrical stimulation to two external electrode pads placed on my skin. Using this stimulator, I was required to exercise the following muscles that are targeted to receive implanted electrodes. The objective was to build the muscles to be prepared for implantation and responsive during surgery.

- Inner thigh muscles on both sides: 45 minutes. The right side surface electrode favors emphasis toward the hamstring. The right hamstring has an implanted electrode that is turned off.

- Gluteus Medius muscles: 45 minutes.

- Right Gluteus Maximus: 45 minutes. It has an implanted electrode that is weak. (No picture is included. I didn't want to moon the world.)

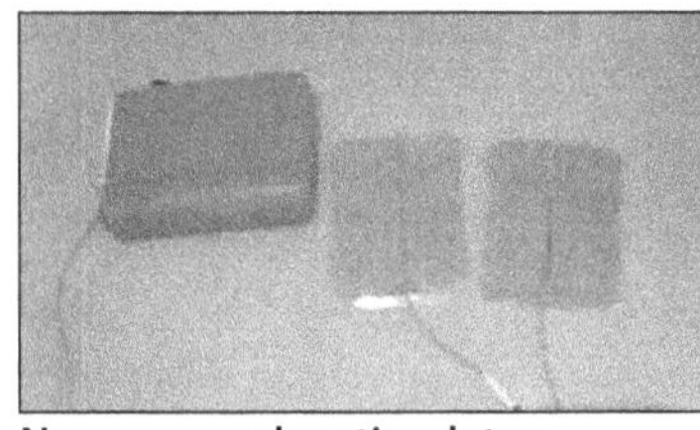
Neuromuscular stimulator

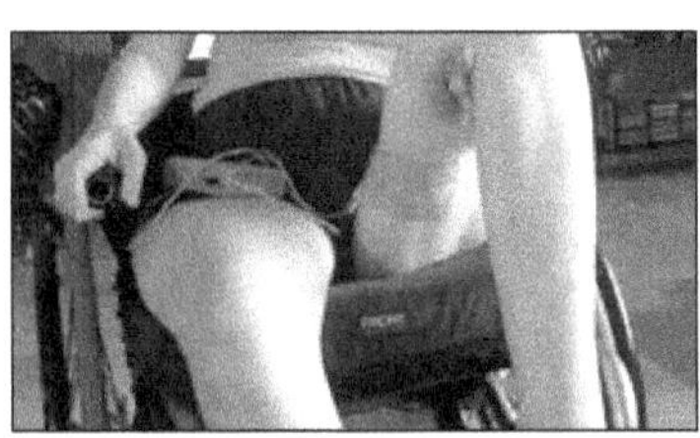
Inner thigh stimulation

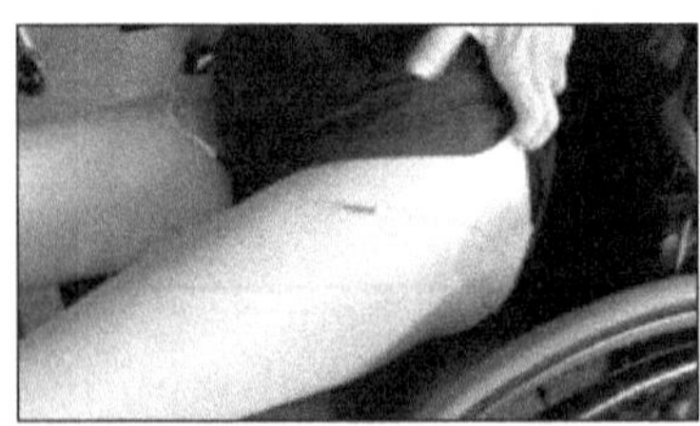
Gluteus medius stimulation

That's a total of 2¼ hours of external stimulation.

Altogether, that is 4¾ hours of exercise per day. All of this is recorded in an exercise log to be given to the research team. Some of this is passive exercise. For instance, while I was writing this, I was exercising my inner thigh and hamstrings. On the other hand, it is not practical to be running around town or sitting in an airport with external electrodes slapped to my skin...imagine getting through airport security! I've discovered that there are certain activities I can do while e-stimming, like writing, reading, or answering emails. But even little movements are not easy. One time, I attempted to make copies while I was e-stimming. Every time the electrodes would turn on, I would get pushed back into my chair. Fitting in the exercise is an adjustment but it is very possible.

Aside from stimulating paralyzed muscles, you really want to be in your best health before going into a long surgery (anticipated duration is 7½ hours). I prepared mentally with relaxation techniques learned from our sailing team sports psychologist. I did cardiovascular conditioning by swimming 28 to 34 laps every three days.

Preparation for surgery is like getting yourself ready for that big competition or regatta. Every piece of the puzzle must fit. It is easy to get overwhelmed by all the components that need to be done but with a daily/weekly plan, it is possible to do my part, as a participant, to contribute to a good outcome.

Being a Conversant Participant

Some of my friends and family worried that all this preparation might be scary to me. But I was ready.

Not long ago, I heard an interview with Dave Matthews, a musician I admire. He made this statement in a different context but it seems appropriate; "It is easy to fear what we don't understand."

Over the past 11 years prior to the upgrade, I had been able to experience the implanted electrode system first-hand, and also follow and be educated on the technological developments over time. I will not pretend to understand all of the engineering and physiology behind the systems, but I understood enough to comprehend the impact. To that end, I wasn't fearful but excited for the upgrade—much like all those people who waited in line for the first iPad.

Being part of a clinical trial requires responsibilities on the part of the participant but also risks. The "Informed Consent" document sets the stage and clearly communicates the risks and responsibilities for taking part in a clinical trial.

I reviewed the main Informed Consent agreement. It's a little like reading documentation for a mortgage and a life insurance policy, all rolled into one. As with mortgage documents (yes, I read ours) it clearly dictates the responsibilities as a participant in full disclosure, such as what I am expected to do over the duration of the trial research, and the time and financial commitments. It also covers the realistic expectation of potential outcomes. The "Risks" section of the informed consent resembles a life insurance policy. It covers many conceivable medical possibilities that can happen in the course of the clinical trial: health risks and what to do if they occur are clearly covered.

A comfort area for me in all of this is knowing I had an "easy out." If I decide that I do not want the implanted system any more, it can be explanted. I run the risk of having scar tissue in the muscles and the skin, but as far as we know, there will be no compromise to the integrity of my central nervous system.

In the end, it is nice to have plenty of time to review the Informed Consent and pose any questions to the research team prior to the surgery date. Upon reflection, this is when it really started to sink in. Then I received a reminder from the airline regarding the upcoming flight and the therapist for the research team reminded me of the countdown to surgery day. *Do I really want to go through with this? Am I ready to take this on?* Those questions entered back into my mind with the final outcome of "yes."

Final Testing

As we drew closer to the surgery date of August 30, more traditional pre-op testing popped up.

Like so many things facing a participant in a clinical trial, nothing is ordinary. The week before surgery I went for pre-op testing at a local hospital where I live in Florida. Since I'm a distant participant, my local doctor follows the progress and I used local medical facilities for some of the preparation. The research team sent me a letter listing the tests needed. It included some typical stuff like blood tests, urine analysis, and chest x-ray, but it also included additional testing like x-rays of the pelvis, knees, and ankles. It's always entertaining to watch the radiology technicians' eyes widen as they see all the hardware in my abdomen from the current system. The experience was actually pleasant. I hadn't been in a hospital for a long while. It was refreshing to be treated as a customer rather than a refugee waiting for rationings.

In addition to the lab tests and x-rays, I had doctor's orders to go sailing. Okay, let me explain. As a member of the 2012 U.S. Paralympic Sailing Team (team website http://racing.ussailing.org/Disabled_Sailing/Paralympics.htm), I spend a lot of time on the water practicing and competing. With this in mind, a concern surfaced about how my body interacts with the boat and adaptive seating system. The research team wanted to understand the pressure points around the hips and thigh areas. With those orders and a Sharpie in hand, we proceeded to the sailing center and hopped in the boat. We marked the edge of the seat on my skin and took photos. We then went sailing and did several common maneuvers on the water and took video of this. The evidence was sent to the research team in Cleveland, to help develop the final surgical plan. So there you have it, I had doctor's orders to go sailing. I was liking this project more and more.

After passing these tests, the research team gave the approval to proceed in the final days prior to surgery. Traveling from Tampa Bay to Cleveland gave me time to reflect on the days passed and those to come. At that point, the hours of exercise began to pay off and I just started to focus on keeping a strong immune system and minimizing risky activities (which is difficult for me to do). The Friday prior to surgery, we met with the surgical team, which also includes the engineers and therapist. This session was to map out the final surgical plan on the skin with a marker and discuss the procedures for the surgery. Sunday evening, I was admitted to the research unit at MetroHealth Medical Center and, yes, more tests. On Monday, August 30, we would begin the long surgery for implanting the system. I would be under anesthesia the entire time and then overcoming the "hangover" for a few days afterwards. If all went well, I'd be on a plane back to Florida on September 3.

This is when all the preparation, the hours of exercising the muscles, and detailed planning come together in this significant milestone. There would be much more work and testing afterwards. But good outcomes here would guide the performance in the future.

Chapter 6: Jen 2.0

While I was is in surgical recovery, the research physical therapist made a posting on my blog on my behalf. The following is in the perspective of the physical therapist.

The Play-by-Play Account

After eight hours, countless pacing time, and lots of concentration, Jen 2.0 has emerged from the operating room at MetroHealth Medical Center. Starting at 0630, Jen was wheeled out of the research unit of the medical center and down into the surgical area for final preparations. There was a bit of chatter while members of the research team poked in to check on their soon-to-be latest technological creation. Then the anesthesiologist went to work.

After the knockout, the surgical team, consisting of four surgeons, two anesthesiologists, six engineers, a very nervous principal investigator, and myself all went to work like an eloquent ballet. We had been over the routines, plans, and procedures many times before this point. But this was to be our premiere.

During the procedure, the 10 electrodes were carefully placed in the planned muscle points. For each placement, approval by the engineer and me (the physical therapist)was required before the surgeons sutured the electrode into the final spot. We began on the backside of the body then flipped her over to complete the system. After placement, the wires for the electrodes were tunneled through the fatty tissue to connector points. From the connector points, the wires weave their way to plug into the implanted receiver. (And you thought the back of your entertainment system looked complicated!)

Patiently in the waiting room was Jen's mom as command cen-

tral. Throughout the surgery, I would emerge to deliver an update to mom. She would then communicate this out. Occasionally, the principal investigator would emerge for more pacing of the floor. After eight hours, the team rolled Jen out of the production room. The job is done successfully. Now it is time for the team to rest and for Jen to slowly get rid of the hangover.

Being Green

It's not easy being green.

Kermit the Frog was on the top of our minds as I was released from the surgical recovery room and moved to the clinical research unit of the hospital. Looking down on my legs, they were green. The antiseptic wash used for surgical preparation turns the skin this green color, it can also protect from infection. With a little anesthesia still in my system, singing Kermit the Frog songs seemed appropriate.

The surgical team ended their long day happy with the outcomes. There seems to be a buzz around here; knowing you are on the verge of something good.

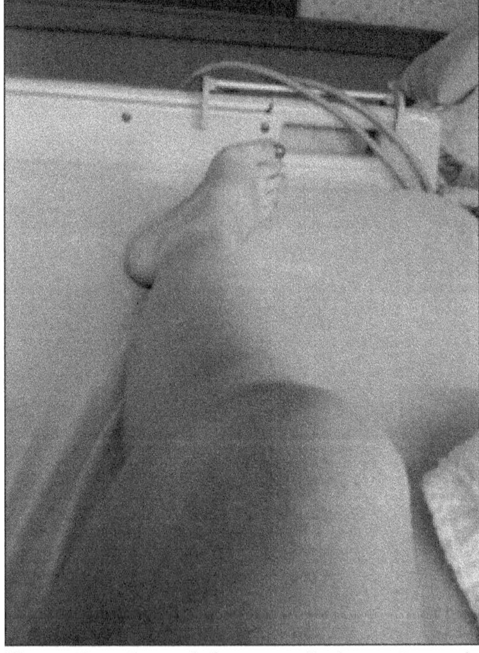

The antiseptic wash from surgical prep turned my leg green.

We had to set the team off to a positive start on surgery day. As the person on the table, I took responsibility for setting the tone (with some help from my sister). On the Friday prior to surgery, they marked on my skin the areas for implant using a purple skin marker. Then, they sent me home (to my sister's house) for the weekend with a skin marker. "Just in case any of the marker started to wash off." Deviously, I seized an opportunity to use the skin marker.

Starting off the day on the surgical table, the research team placed me on my belly to start the surgery on my backside. Over the weekend, my sister and I left a message on my gluteus maximus to the research team; "Kiss Me." We also made a smiley face on my belly button. We thought it would at least provide some comic relief for the long day of surgery.

Apparently the anesthesia cocktail used to knock me out, aka margarita on the rocks with salt, was not so bad. The transition from knockout to wakeup was smooth. Amazing, particularly since we planned to have me out with a hangover for at least 24 hours. Post surgery, I was awake pretty quick and yappy as ever on the move from the recovery room to the clinical research unit. This is the nursing unit where I spent the next five days getting back to normal.

If there is any place to be after a long surgery, it is the CRU (Clinical Research Unit). My favorite nurses were there. Most were there when I had my first implant in 1999; some retired and came back. Coming here was a bit of a reunion. This nursing unit focuses on research. The team is extremely skilled, they deliver comfort when you need it, and they make you laugh when you are in pain. Of course, homemade cookies from mom didn't hurt either. (Although the residents ate most of those.)

Otherwise, recovery was very similar to that from any big surgical procedure.

- Progress from Jell-O and soup to solid foods (well hospital food)

- Vitals (blood pressure, temperature, pulse) and rolling every two hours

- Breathing exercises to restore lung capacity

- Visits from residents at 3 am

- Shedding of needles and IV tubes

Then there is the glue man.

They used sutures and skin glue to close all the incisions from surgery. The glue, much like super glue (but don't try this at home) seals the wound to help protect from infections. A resident came in afterwards with a glue stick in hand to re-seal all the incisions. Just like super glue, it can't touch anything until it dries. Otherwise, I might have been glued to the bed!

The days moved fast. Day three was the first time back in my wheelchair. Within about 10 minutes I said, "Let's go for a stroll." The hospital room gets small after a few days. This was the time to transition home and understand the restrictions of activity. We took x-rays of the system within the body. Testing was done with a scope to make sure the system was intact.

My cheering sections on the Internet—besides my blog, I was on Facebook, Plaxo, and Linkedin plus plain old email—proved to be very comforting. They made the process much easier. I was very grateful to have them all out there. Now, I was back to my green body and transitioning home.

Some day you'll find it, the rainbow connection.
The lovers, the dreamers and me.

Chapter 7: Returning Home

One of my friends had messaged me, "Home is where the healing process begins," and there is a lot of truth to that.

Sometimes I think that hospitals deliberately try to make some amenities miserable just so we are encouraged to go home. Take for instance food. After surgery, it is common to transition to a liquid diet consisting of Jell-O, chicken broth, etc. But I was sent chicken broth for every day thereafter—high-sodium chicken broth.

This is when family came to the rescue. After my sister got a whiff of a salmon patty that looked like some mystery meat you'd get at a fast food joint and smelled like the dumpster out back, she brought me lunch the next day. Vegetables—beloved fresh vegetables—never tasted so good. Vegetables, not overcooked or smothered in unknown white sauce, constituted my biggest meal while in the hospital. And on top of that she brought fruit, not from a can or stagnant in corn syrup, but fresh fruit. My mom followed suit the next day. Then my first day home, friends brought over a homemade quiche. Those were my first tastes of the comforts of home.

Advice for Leaving the Hospital

On the trip back to Florida, I was accompanied by my mom and it was pretty uneventful but with a few lessons learned.

First, don't forget your discharge papers. I was so excited to get home that I completely forgot to do the proper procedures for discharge. Thank God for cell phones, fax machines, and email.

Next, be straightforward with airport security. Going through airport security is never easy for people with disabilities (not that it's a piece of cake for people *without* disabilities). I had notes on letterhead from every organization involved in this research project with one in particular explaining the dos and don't for post surgery recovery. As a security agent pulled me aside, I handed them the letters right away, then worked with them to get through the process.

Finally, take the pain medications before getting on the flight. I'm not a person who takes pain medication. Not because I'm a "tough guy" but I hate how they make me feel and cloud my thinking. Again, excited to go home, I forgot to take the hospital-issued Tylenol. In my pocket book I only had one Tylenol, which wore off half way down to Florida. By the time we departed the aircraft, I was in pain and very punchy. Fortunately, my mom has the patience of a saint and I was lucky she didn't smack me upside the head.

We made it back. To minimize transfers, we arranged my adapted ramp van for wheelchair tie-downs and my mom drove us from the airport to our home.

The biggest comfort of home came that evening in the form of a full night of sleep without interruptions at wee hours of the morning *and* in my own bed. Ahhh!!! The comforts of home!

Adjusting to Home

Okay, so maybe home isn't so comfy? Have you ever entered your home and it just seems different? Maybe you came home after a long vacation or after losing a loved one; for that matter you came home after being in the hospital for several days or weeks. It's not that your home changed. The fact of the matter is *you* changed. You are looking at familiar surroundings through different eyes. This feeling is captured so well in the movie "Murderball." (If you haven't seen it and you live or work with people living with spinal cord injuries, it is a movie worth watching.) In the movie there is a scene when a man, new to living with a spinal cord injury, goes home from the rehabilitation hospital for the first time. You can see it in his eyes. He has changed but his home has not.

The good news is we have a cunning ability to adapt. We take on this adaptation without even thinking about it. Along with the welcoming comforts of home after returning from Cleveland, I had to adapt to the new restrictions in my familiar home. Understand that I live in a fairly wheelchair-accessible home (with the exception of our kitchen, which has not been adapted yet). There is an adjustment period to my surroundings given the instructions from the research team.

For the next 5½ weeks, I was put on "restricted activity." That meant:

- Only four transfers per day
- No strenuous activity
- No bending at the hip more than 90 degrees
- No bending forward in the wheelchair, use reachers to retrieve items on the floor

That may not seem like much but think about it. Two transfers are taken up each day for getting in and out of bed. A reacher is needed every time I dropped something on the floor. Many daily activities require bending, like feeding the cats, putting on shoes, filling the dishwasher, etc. I'm not complaining but just pointing out the adjustments needed that you don't realize until you are in the situation.

As a result, I adapted the "different" to feel familiar again. Thanks to the help of my mom and Tim, this adjustment was easier. Those old reachers were strategically placed in every room of the house. Items used on a daily basis migrated from low storage to higher. I became more careful not to drop anything on the floor. Transfers in and out of the wheelchair were planned for every day and it became a game of tradeoffs. Driving was out of the question; that would take up two transfers right there.

Choosing days to shower was also an adjustment. Speaking of bathing, any cruiser out there knows that freshwater showers can be a luxury. I've had my time on long trips aboard a cruising sailboat, coming ashore after several days and taking that long awaited hot shower. After more than a week and with some green tint still lingering on my skin, I really enjoyed my first shower post surgery.

Now, that is a feeling all too familiar.

Managing 15

"Two, four, six, eight, nine—okay we need to find six more." Words spoken from my local physician, as he shook his head like a speechless parent discovering his child just got a tattoo. A couple weeks after returning home, I met with my local doctor to observe the progress of the incisions as they healed. I think he was in a little disbelief by seeing so many incisions, but when I started to tell him of potential functional gains like trunk control and standing stability, he understood the payoff.

Fifteen is the total count of incisions from the surgery. There are 10 incisions for each electrode, one for the implanted receiver, and four for the connector points. Connector points are "pass-throughs" for the wires routed to the implanted receiver. The incisions are closed with internal sutures and skin glue externally. The skin glue was beginning to peel off and expose the scars resulting from the surgery. Each time one was exposed, it got a daily treatment of vitamin E. As it turns out the fabulous 15 were healing well.

But I have to admit, I would look down at my abdomen and wonder. It's hard to believe 12 years ago when I was first injured, one scar was such a concern. At the time, I did everything I could to conceal that one scar on the back of my neck. That one scar was the result of the vertebrae fusion surgery after my accident. I wore collared shirts, neck scarves with blouses, and countless turtlenecks just to conceal that one scar. Now, I have 13 scars from the first implanted system and 15 from the most recent upgrade, for a total of 28. But those 28 are mostly concealed by everyday clothing. Unless I wear a bikini (and I don't plan to do so any time soon), the scars are not even noticeable and are mostly hidden.

I've become acutely aware of the image industry filled with plastic surgeons, tattoo artists, anti-aging creams, and scar-reduction potions. As it turns out, advice from a knowledgeable researcher in the area of wound healing said that good old vitamin E or retinol cream can do a good job of promoting skin healing. My 28 scars tell a story. Who needs tattoos? These scars are my body art.

Missing the System

It had been over four weeks since the surgery to implant the upgraded system. More apparent, it had been over four weeks since I last used the old implanted system. It had been that long since I last stood out of my wheelchair, used back electrodes for trunk control, or exercised the endurance fibers in the implanted muscles.

Okay, I can adjust to not being able to stand for a few months. That adjustment is easy because in the back of my mind, it is a short-term sacrifice for a long-term gain. Not being able to stand or use the trunk control features causes some daily living inconveniences. That adjustment period was eerily similar to what I experienced when I was first introduced to life as a wheelchair user. In the end, the inconvenient sacrifices were not as traumatic knowing that in the near future I would have the capability back and hopefully with more function.

The real noticeable change is physiological; those changes that are not obvious but creep into your daily life and have a significant impact. My internal systems were not performing as they usually did. Things like urinary and fecal tracks, digestion, and circulation all changed. As a person with an incomplete spinal cord injury who has motor paralysis but retained sensation, my rear end and back became sore from sitting in the wheelchair for most of the day. Not being able to exercise those muscles and the ongoing threat of a pressure sore constantly lingered in the back of my mind. The biggest change, however, was the increased spasticity.

Spasticity is common among people living with central nervous system disorders. It is described as an ongoing level or sudden burst of contraction of a muscle, with decreased ability to volitionally control the muscle contraction, and increased resistance felt on passive stretch. Contractions can be so strong that people experience extreme rigidity or get tossed out of a wheelchair. There are many ways to manage this condition. The most common in the U.S. is a pharmaceutical solution.

When I was first injured, I tried that solution. Just like pain medications, I could not function productively while using a drug that has a base as a muscle relaxer. Over the years, I had used stretching and electrical stimulation to keep the condition under control. While in this recovery stage, stretching my lower extremities was restricted and use of surface electrical stimulation was permitted only below the knee. This helped but is still not sufficient to keep spasticity from rearing its ugly head.

At this point, psychologically and functionally, I had adjusted for the short term without using the system. With less than two weeks to go until the limited activity stage would be behind me, the return to being active and the moment of turning on the new system was in sight. But more significantly in the short term, my body had missed the system.

One More Week

There was one more week to go of restricted activity. At that point, my incisions had healed, the skin glue was off and I was exercising with light arms weights. I became restless to start being active again.

It would be one more week before we could also turn on the system for the first time since the surgery. When the research team implanted the electrodes on August 30, for each electrode they would place it in the muscle tissue, and then turn on the stimulation to test the contraction of the muscle against the placement of the electrode. When they found the optimal contraction, the surgeons secured the electrode in place and left the electrode to rest and the tissue to grow around it.

When we would finally turn on the system thc following week it did not mean I would be standing out of my wheelchair. If any researcher had told me that after six weeks of sedentary recovery, I would be standing and moving around instantly, then that same person is probably selling snake oil too.

The following week, I was scheduled to meet with members of the research team in the laboratory at MetroHealth Medical Center. We would spend several hours testing each electrode individually, a process called profiling. Then the therapist would issue an exercise regime for the next eight weeks. The regime is designed to slowly build the muscle fibers (both strength and endurance fibers) using the implanted electrodes. Just as body builders slowly add weights to the barbells and marathon runners slowly add miles to their running routine, I slowly increased weights and repetitions for each muscle group. There is no instant gratification. Just as I learned in rehab after my initial injury, recovery is a slow process. Instead of focusing on daily progress, it is more productive to focus on the long-term goal.

In the meantime, I have one more week with these limitations. As I'm looking forward to turning on the new system, Tim and I will celebrate our anniversary. We will be remembering a magical day when we committed our wedding vows while I was using the original system.

Chapter 8: Flipping the Switch

After months of anticipation, in October 2010 we flipped the switch on the new system. But it was not as easy as flipping a switch to turn on a light. Oh no. It was much more involved. Add in the complexity of the human body, and you have hours of tweaking.

I traveled up to Cleveland on Wednesday, October 13 with lab time scheduled for Thursday and Friday. Filled with excitement, it was hard to contain myself. Sleeping that night was difficult; like a kid on Christmas Eve waiting for St. Nick to arrive. I resorted to the relaxation techniques taught by the sailing team's sports psychologist. I grabbed my headphones and listened to some music. Ironically, the same song that I listened to before going into surgery played that night; John Mayer, "Why Georgia," with a line that resonates with me: *Am I living it right?*

Coming to Cleveland is always a homecoming. Not just the visits with family and friends, but after working with the FES Center for 11 years it's like entering a Norman Rockwell Thanksgiving. Aside from the work we have to do, the days are filled with hugs, welcomes, and catch-up conversations. Our physical therapist keeps me in order.

We had two days scheduled in the laboratory. On day one we got right to work. This is a smaller team than the army we had for the surgery. The team in the lab consisted of the physical therapist, two engineers, and the principal investigator, although he keeps a comfortable distance to allow the other members to do their work. With some baggy shorts on, I transferred onto a therapy mat with an adjacent table filled with coils, external control units, and recording papers.

Electrode Profiling

Our first rule of order was profiling. This is a procedure used to test each individual electrode to understand the threshold and saturation points. What does that mean? In layman's terms, we are trying to find the setting, when an active electrode produces a visible contraction of the stimulated muscle and also to find the point when the maximum stimulation is tolerable and does not produce an adverse effect. Current (in milliamps), pulse width (in microseconds) and frequency (in hertz) are all electrical parameters that can be tweaked to create an optimal muscle contraction. We perform this testing for each of the new channels. The physical therapist is watching any movement of the muscle and any overflow to other muscles. This is graded according to a standard rating scale of 0 to 5, with 0 corresponding to no movement and 5 corresponding to normal function/strength.

During the testing, the engineer is working his magic with the external control unit, pressing buttons so fast that it sounded like he was sending a message in Morse Code. For the original system, this process took about an hour. For the new system, we scheduled three hours. It just was not enough. Maybe it was the interruptions, the side conversations, the testing of new electrode combinations, or additional troubleshooting. By mid-day, we were not nearly done. We did confirm that one-hour profiling sessions are a thing of the past.

The highlight of the profiling session was the use of the new cuff electrodes implanted around the femoral nerve to control the quad muscles. Only a few people have been implanted with this technology on the femoral nerve. The cuff electrode has four channels in each electrode and we are able to test each individual channel to see how that specific stimulation impacts the group of quad muscles.

While I was lying on my back on the mat, we placed a bolster under my knees. Here we turned on the channels in the cuff electrodes and watched how the stimulation would contract the quad muscle to extend the knee and straighten the leg. We first contracted the quad using the original epimysial electrode in the quad. It would straighten the knee and lift the foot off the mat, but there was minimal strength; the therapist was able to push the leg back down with one finger. We then contracted the quad muscle using the new cuff electrode. My leg straightened out with full force and the therapist graded the movement with a 5 for full extension and strength.

Watching the leg kick out is a visual I still love today. And apparently, research team members like it too. During the long profiling process the Principal Investigator kept coming back to the mat to inquire about the cuff electrodes, like a kid on a long car trip asking, "Are we there yet?" Then the chief surgeon came in and wanted to see the "new quads" and then the center director came in to see it too. My kicks were so good, I have visions of becoming a football place kicker, or maybe a Rockette.

After profiling, there were additional hours on the dynamometer machine to, yes, test the cuff electrodes. Now dubbed "pulse pumping," the experiments sought to find a more effective and efficient way to test the electrodes and further understand how fatigue changes with multiple pulses while varying the resting time. I can't tell you how many hours I have spent on this machine but it is a necessity not just for research but to help find the optimum system performance.

On day two we were back on the mat to tweak more contraction combinations for functional performance. Since I was unable to stand yet, the functional uses of the system included trunk control in the wheelchair and gluts shift for pressure relief. Once we completed the tweaking, the engineer took the external control unit back to his office to do some final programming. Meanwhile, the therapist reviewed the next phase of the research protocol, the exercise phase, which is designed to slowly build the strength and endurance fibers of the implanted muscles. There is not only an instruction sheet describing each exercise, but also a daily exercise log. Even though they are capturing usage data in the external unit, they still want to understand user compliance.

After about 20 minutes, the engineer emerged with a Universal External Control Unit (UECU) and an exercise plan. I was back to the mat to test all the exercise patterns. Here I per-

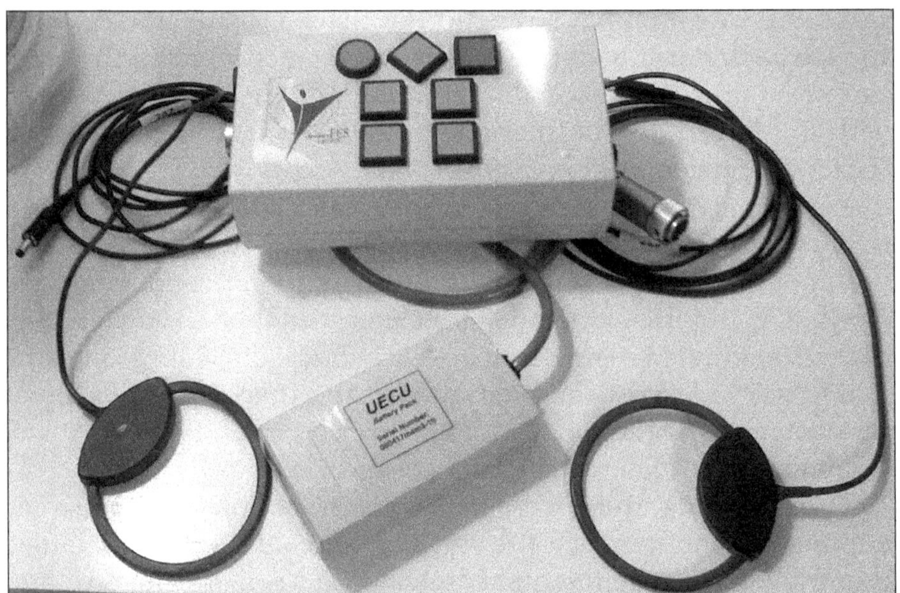

The Universal External Control Unit

formed one set of each exercise while the therapist watched for any adverse reactions. Once we were happy with the exercise patterns, we went back on the dynamometer machine for more testing. By the end of two days in the lab, my body was exhausted. The amount of physical exertion is deceiving.

What did we learn with all this testing? First, we discovered the proper settings to begin the exercise phase. Second, we found one channel on the cuff electrode that was not providing the same quality of contraction as the others, which is to be expected. That's the whole reason for having multiple contacts within the cuff in the first place. We were not exactly sure why that was happening; it might have been that the contact was simply over connective tissue or a part of the nerve that wouldn't cause a muscle contraction. We would watch it closely and retest it on the next visit. Regardless, the remaining channels provided super strong contractions and we were confident that I could stand without this problem child. Finally, we learned that we needed to schedule more lab time for testing and profiling.

They sent me home with a case full of toys. We had a UECU with customized exercise patterns, multiple coils, auxiliary batteries, and battery charger—and a mission to start exercising. Resting time was over. It was now my job to get up and exercise. The exercises were necessary to build up muscle strength and endurance in preparation for the first stand using the upgraded system. We now were entering eight weeks of exercising and monitoring of the system. Body builders have nothing on me.

Delivering the Power

Some of my geekier friends asked if more ports could be added to the UECU to accommodate a cell phone, computer, and USB drive. Okay, so we have a world of multitasking. At this point, I was like a two-year-old learning how to stand. I decided that I should stay focused on the task at hand.

As people integrate their lives with technology, they become more power hungry. Going through the airport one day, I couldn't help but notice the gathering of people huddled around power supply stations. We even have portals under the airplane seats. As we become more mobile, we rely more on battery power.

These inquiries touch on a key issue for so many devices are implanted into the human body. How do we power them up? Today, there are pacemakers and spinal cord stimulation systems with implanted batteries. This works for devices that only require a very low current. For a system like mine, the need for power is too great for the currently available implantable battery technology. Therefore, the power source is external.

To power up the implanted standing system, the UECU, which houses the rechargeable batteries, transmits power via high level radio frequency (RF) signals through the coil and to the implanted receiver inside my body. This is evident when I touch the **On** button of the UECU and I get a little jolt of power. As long as the UECU is on and the coil is coupled with the receiver, then there is power going to it. Like talk time on your cell phone, the system draws more power when it is stimulating than when it is idle. Use duration for one battery charge is approximately 2 hours. In other words, I can get 2 hours of stimulation without recharging the batteries. At this point in the exer-

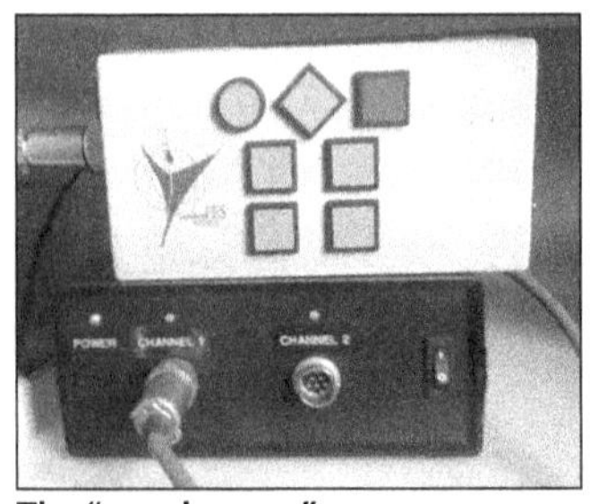

The "car charger"

cise regime, I am stimulating for about 2 hours per day. This is why I also carry a small auxiliary battery with me.

Recharging the batteries is not as mobile as the small charger coils for a cell phone. Oh no, it is much bigger. Dubbed by Tim, the "car charger" is a big black box weighing in at about 5 pounds. The reason the battery charger is so big is that the FDA requires several safety measures. Some of these measures are in place to allow me to receive stimulation while the UECU is connected to the "car charger."

The system is power hungry and the addition of a laptop or cell phone connection is not feasible. So, don't expect to see holiday lights flashing from my head while I am using the UECU. That would have to be part of a different research project.

Early Observations

Four weeks had now passed in the exercise phase of the research protocol. A total of eight weeks were required before I could start to use the system for standing. What did I notice since I started using the implanted electrodes to build the tissue in my paralyzed muscles?

Here are three key observations.

One of the daily exercises is **Leg Lifts**. Here, I use the stimulation to lift the legs against gravity by extending the knee. The exercise is designed to build the quadriceps muscle group in the front of the thigh. After two weeks of exercise with no weights, the therapist gave me clearance to add ankle weights until I observed fatigue. Well, I progressively added one pound each day. I reached nine pounds with no fatigue. I either had to buy more weights or start with more repetitions. To give you some perspective, before the recent upgrade surgery, I could perform leg lifts using stimulation from the original system and maxed out from fatigue at three pounds. I was now at nine pounds and potentially seeking more. Conclusively, the quadriceps muscles are building nicely. This muscle group is extremely important to be able to stand out of the wheelchair and also to remain standing.

Another observation from using the new implanted system for those first few weeks concerned the coupling of the external coil to the new receiver. Coupling just means to align the external coil to the implanted receiver to properly deliver the signal from the UECU to the receiver. If the coil and receiver are not coupled, the implanted system will not receive the stimulation.

With the upgrade, I now have two receivers implanted into the abdominal area. The one on the left side is the original IRS-8 and the one on the right side is the new IST-16. After using the IRS-8 for so many years, I know the best place to tape the coil to the skin over the receiver. It is almost automatic like popping in contact lenses every morning. However, I found that the placement of the coil over the IST-16 was still not perfected. I was still trying to find the optimum placement on a daily basis and how to rotate the coil around the skin for the best comfort and a good signal. I attributed this to user adaptation since each user has a different anatomy. This exercise phase was truly the time to figure this one out!

The third key observation in this exercise phase had to do with the change in the **Extends All** exercise. The **Extends All** pattern is designed to build the endurance fibers in the implanted muscles. This exercise is performed by lying on my back with the legs out straight. All of the implanted muscles contract using stimulation at the same time for 10 seconds followed by 10 seconds of rest. This pattern continues for 60 minutes with minimal motion of the legs. I had this exercise pattern with the original eight electrode system and used it frequently to control my spasticity. Now with the upgraded system and more electrodes the same exercise pattern uses more muscles. Boy, do I feel it. Near the end of the 60 minutes, I am thirsty for water, begin to feel fatigue, and become warm from the workout.

Still, these exercises built up my muscles and I progressed to exercising two hours per day. However, this is no substitute for exercising other parts of the body. Even though I was getting great movement, circulation, and stimulation, I still needed to pay attention to cardiovascular exercise and workout of the upper body. A key area that tends to be overlooked when working with people with paralysis is that we need a full body workout just like those with able bodies. We need to exercise our moving limbs, our cardiovascular system *and* our paralyzed limbs.

UECU Swap

The UPS man strutted up our driveway to the front porch where he was greeted by our muscovy duck, who had nested under our jasmine bush. He dropped the hard black case by the door and shouted through the open window, "UPS!" I made my way to the front door just in time to give him a wave for the day. This routine happened every two weeks.

Since bringing the UECU home in mid-October, we started a ritual called the "UECU Swap." For this exercise phase, the swap occurs every two weeks. The main purpose of this swap is to progress the exercise patterns to work on endurance to prepare for standing. Just as physical trainers will add repetitions to a routine, the therapists and engineers were adjusting my exercise patterns. For instance, the exercise pattern **Extends All** delivers a low level of stimulation to all the electrodes; oscillating on and off for an hour duration. The purpose is to build the endurance fibers in the stimulated muscles. As I progressed over time, they increased the stimulation time. For example, the pattern changed at one point from 10 seconds of stimulation followed by 10 seconds of rest to 15 seconds of stimulation followed by 10 seconds of rest.

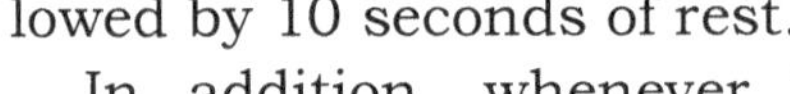

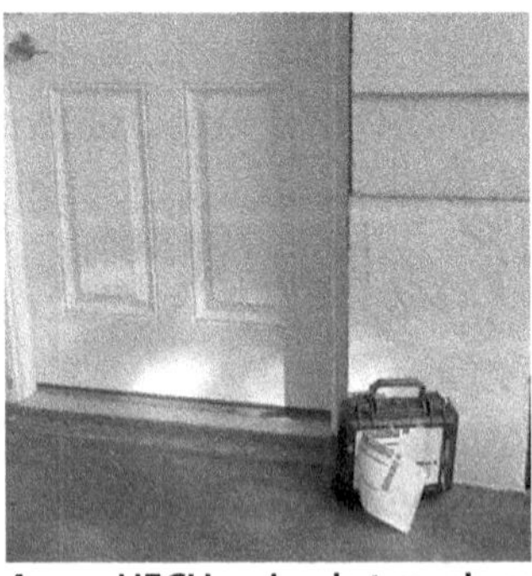

A new UECU arrived at my door by UPS every two weeks.

In addition, whenever I used the UECU, it recorded usage data. The usage data is basically recording the patterns that I used with the UECU. For instance, it not only recorded how many sets of leg lifts I was doing, but also the date and time that I performed that specific exercise. They need this data for analysis later in the clinical study. In addition to the usage data collected by the UECU, I personally recorded the repetitions and duration of the exercises, along with the weights that I was using, on the paper exercise log. While the UECU can monitor the amount or time of exercise, it can't record the amount of pounds used for ankle weights and it can't record if I am watching David Letterman or Conan O'Brien while exercising. But it records enough so the research team knew if and when the exercises were being performed.

Every two weeks, I received a fresh box. It contained a UECU with amended patterns and a clean data log. I returned the UECU that I had been using, which holds the data for the previous two weeks. It is packed up into the hard black case along with the exercise logs. I scheduled a UPS pick up and set it on the front porch. Then I would await the afternoon greeting through my front window, "UPS!"

Back in the Saddle Again

As I rounded out the final few weeks of the exercise phase, I reached yet another milestone in this long process. I was back sailing...okay other watersports too.

As I learned from this experience, the human body takes a long time to heal. It truly is all relative. But from the perspective of the person eagerly waiting to meet the healing milestone, it takes a very long time. And the final days are even longer, like those last few days before Christmas. Six weeks after surgery, I was released to daily transfer counts, the ability to lean and bend over and regular daily activity. However, I was still restricted from any watersports. Finally, almost three months after my surgery in August, I was released from the restriction on watersports.

I fully understand why the research team decided to extend this limitation but it did not make the wait any easier. The extra months allowing the body to heal and the tissue to grow around the new implanted devices helps to ensure that when I start banging my body around, the hardware should remain anchored.

For the average person living in cooler climates, this constraint may not seem like a big deal. For me, however, it was a long time off the water. Living in Florida, the fall and winter seasons mark the perfect time to get outdoors. Canoeing and kayaking is great that time of the year. It also marked the start of the sailboat racing season in the South. I was a member of the U.S. Sailing Team. But I had been restricted from the sport I love and from valuable practice time as we geared up for the U.S. Paralympics trials, which would determine the team to represent Team USA at the 2012 Paralympics Games in London.

My teammate, Jean-Paul or JP, had been extremely patient. We had taken the time to do the much needed boat work and administrative tasks that also go along with campaigning for the Paralympic Games.

Getting back on the water truly marked the end of the recovery phase. I was finally back to my normal activities. I was back on the water the day after Thanksgiving with the weeks following filled with team training camps and com-

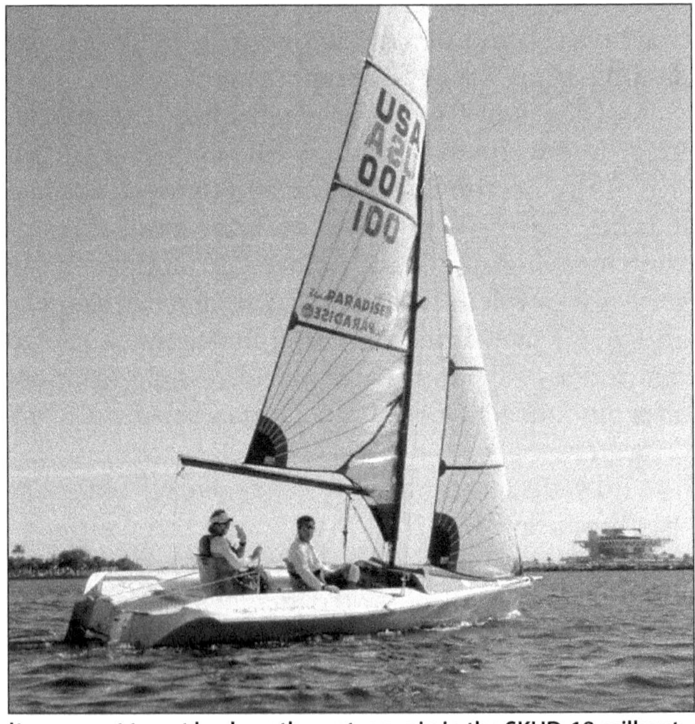

It was great to get back on the water again in the SKUD-18 sailboat.

peting in the U.S. Disabled Sailing National Championship, http://championships.ussailing.org/Adult/USDisabledChampionship.htm

I was like a kid who gets to eat Fruit Loops at her grandparent's house while at home the parents only allow organic granola—I was gorging in excitement. After being prohibited from sailing for three months, I was back on the water and in the saddle again.

Chapter 9: Rejoining the Upright World

After four full days in the Cleveland lab, we had many hours of testing, discoveries, and some surprises. December is not the ideal time to travel from Tampa Bay to Cleveland, but in this case it was a good exception. A few days before making the trek north, the headline news was about a snowstorm crippling the Midwest. The storm was expected to hit the Cleveland area on the same day of my scheduled arrival. Regardless, the flight was not delayed, let alone cancelled. Putting on every layer of clothing I own, I made my way to Cleveland. We landed with the white fluffy snow coming down as the flight attendant welcomed us to Cleveland. My Mom would pick me up at the airport and I would stay at my sister's home. This was the beginning of four stacked days with the research team. I was counting on my eight weeks of exercise to pay off.

Day One

As I was getting ready for my mom to pick me up for our drive to MetroHealth Medical Center, my sister rapped on the door. "You know, over 400 area schools are closed due to the snow storm. You may want to see if the research team will cancel." Yeah, welcome to Cleveland and the signature lake effect snow. Images of delayed lab progress, treacherous driving conditions and freezing temperatures started flying around in my head. With that, I started calling members of the research team. The diehard Ohioans were making their way into the lab and they were expecting me to be there too. In the end, the roads were not bad and we were able to start the first day of testing with only an hour delay.

After the ritual hugs of hello, we made our way back to the

lab for the first priority at hand, profiling. This is the process of testing each individual channel of the system. The testing is done on a therapy mat. The first channels to test are those in the quadriceps. To do this, I lay supine on the mat and we placed a bolster under my knee. We then connect the coils to a UECU programmed specifically for testing. The engineer operates this UECU, dubbed the "Morse Code Box" because the engineer clicks the buttons so fast that it sounds like Morse Code. We tested the channels for the right side first. The engineer turned on one channel and began to turn up the juice and the leg began to extend. He got to 200 milliamps and the knee dropped down and got weaker.

The therapist asked to repeat the process, while I held my breath hoping that nothing was wrong with the system. The second time around showed the same results and the third round the same. We stopped, perplexed. The engineer looked down and said, "I'll be right back." He rushed back to his office to reload the programs into the test UECU. When he arrived, we plugged everything back in and Voila! It worked. Apparently, the programs did not download correctly into the test unit. We repeated the test on the same channel and it was all okay.

During the first profile in October, we discovered one channel in the cuff electrode that was not responding. That channel had been turned off for the past eight weeks. At this point, it was time to turn it back on to test the mystery channel. To our surprise, when we turned the channel on, it performed as it was designed to do; it contracted the right quadricep. With a few more tests we were now able to use this channel. This was probably one of the most eventful profiling sessions we have had.

With the profiling complete and still on the mat, we began to play around with the trunk control patterns. This pattern uses three sets of electrodes. Those implanted in the gluteus maximus, quadradus, and erector spinae. The key thing that we were trying to find is the best settings to get a balanced sitting posture without spillover to other muscles and a comfortable contraction. Once we found the proper settings, I was off the mat and onto the dynamometer machine.

The dynamometer machine is a testing unit. I have spent many hours on this machine and my log time will not end any time soon. The main goal is to test the channels in the cuff electrodes. The lead engineer in this area of research is trying to understand the channels that produce the strongest contraction, the setting where spillover to other muscles begins and what oscillation patterns he can develop to decrease fatigue in the coveted quadriceps muscle group.

After a lunch break, we were back in the lab. The afternoon holds the climax to the eight weeks of exercise, the first stand with the new system. We tested a few more patterns before the initial attempt. Cameras were in place and the parallel bars were reassembled. “Okay, are we all ready to stand?” The therapist is the one in charge and she makes the call “Now!”

I pressed the little green button to activate the system, the muscles contracted and I stood straight up. I towered over her as she remained seated on the PT square stool guarding my knees. That stand felt so good! But after only 1½ minutes, my left knee began to buckle as a sign of fatigue and the PT gave the command to sit. I tried not to wear the emotion of disappointment on my face, but it obviously showed. Attempting to provide words of comfort, the principal investigator said, “Jen, you haven’t stood in four months. Remember your first stand (11 years ago) was less than that.” That effort to cheer me up didn’t work. Now we needed to troubleshoot. We did a few more

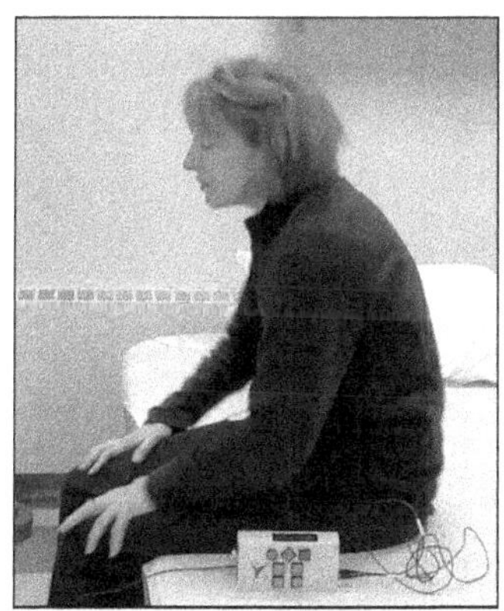
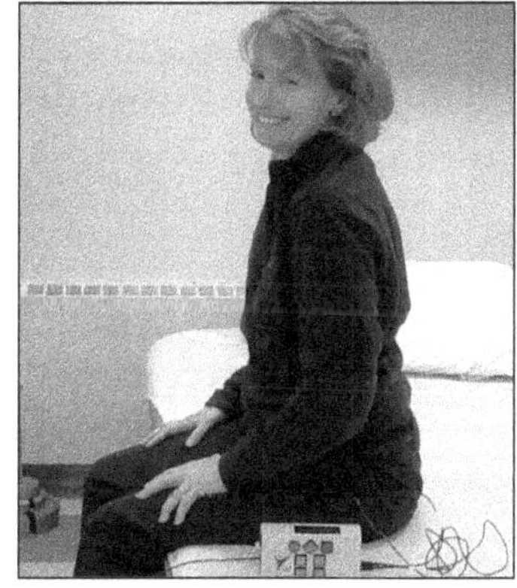

Trunk stability with stimulation off (left) and on (right)

short stands and observed that I am standing with all my weight on the left leg and the right leg was off the ground. We called it a day knowing that we'd have a few more days to troubleshoot the system. If it was easy, then it wouldn't be science.

Day Two

On the second day, my mom and I met members of the research team at the Louis Stokes VA Hospital. We were at the VA Hospital to run several tests using the new trunk control patterns. One particular test was to see if the trunk patterns will assist with wheelchair propulsion. The therapist set up a course around an inpatient ward. The experiment was to propel the wheelchair as far as I could within a six-minute duration. We did this without stimulation, with full trunk stimulation, and with reduced trunk stimulation. We ran two tests with each scenario.

Talk about getting my workout for the day. I was wheeling as fast as I could around the nurses' ward while the therapist ran/walked along side me to help clear the way. By the time we did the third test, we had our cheering sections at various parts of the course. I almost ran over a nurse and kept the janitorial team on their toes. While still at the VA, we met up with other members of the research team to test ramp patterns and pressure-relief patterns.

For the afternoon, we made our way back to MetroHealth Medical Center for more testing on the dynamometer machine. We all agreed to stay late in order to complete the tests. The engineer would take the data and crunch the numbers over the evening in order to be armed with information to help us troubleshoot the standing pattern during the next day.

Day Three

Halfway through the four day schedule and we still had a lot of work to accomplish. We started day three by meeting our dynamometer engineer, who crunched the numbers over the evening. I was back on the machine to start the day. For these tests, we experimented with various combinations of oscillating the channels in the cuff electrodes to reduce fatigue. We tried several different combinations. One pattern was oscillating between three different channels. My upper thigh looked like it was on a massage chair with muscles rolling on and off from the contractions.

Testing completed, it was time for the DEXA scan. A research team nurse escorted me down to the Clinical Research Unit (CRU) for the test. The CRU is the special area in MetroHealth Medical Center where I did inpatient recovery after the implant surgery in August. Here I was able to revisit some of my favorite nurses. The DEXA scan uses laser technology to scan the body and analyze bone density. For people living with chronic spinal cord injuries, brittle bones and osteoporosis is a common health risk. Being 12 years post injury, I was expecting bad news. To my surprise, it was quite the opposite. The results from scanning my pelvic area showed that my bone density is within normal range for an able-body woman of my same age, height, and weight. Yes, that's right. After 12 years of being a wheelchair user and an electrical stimulation user, my bone density was normal. Unbelievable!

With results in hand, we headed back to the lab for an afternoon of tweaking the standing parameters. To give ourselves a reality check, the engineer loaded the original standing patterns that I was using before the implant surgery in August. I stood with the original eight-channel system and the physical therapist said, "I am not impressed." We then turned back to the standing pattern with the new system. I stood and she said, "I'm still not impressed." Now, we had some problem solving to do.

The first challenge was to get me standing on both feet. On day one, we discovered that I was weight bearing on only one leg. The suggested solution from the research team was that the glut medius on the left side was pulling the hip up on the right side. We gradually reduced the glut medius on the left until the right hip lowered and I was standing solidly on both feet. First problem solved.

The next standing challenge was to figure out why my left quad muscles were fatiguing within only 1½ minutes. One theory pointed to the stimulation of the quadriceps muscle group. With the new system, I was standing with five channels of stimulation on each quad; four channels in the new cuff electrodes and one epimysial electrode from the original system. We thought that we were over-stimulating the muscles, which was causing a fast fatigue in standing performance. We used the data from the dynamometer testing to help us.

We first turned off the original epimysial electrode. Not much difference. The engineer reviewed the data and found the one channel in each cuff electrode that provided the strongest muscle contraction. From there the standing pattern was programmed to stand on just one of the five channels in the quad. I stood for seven minutes. We were on to something. We then programmed to stand with one channel and tweaked the second strongest channel without any spillover to the other muscles in the group. We turned down the stimulation to 50 percent. It worked. I stood for only a few minutes but we knew the problem was solved.

The final challenge for the afternoon was to test the swing through gait. This is using the walker to pull the body off the ground, then swing both legs forward in order to move around short distances. We found that my right hip was flexing and the right leg was swinging far forward and I was barely landing on the heel. We began to test the stimulated muscles to find the culprit that was flexing the hip. The tests pointed us to the right back electrode. We gradually turned the stimulation down. It reduced the problem but did not solve it completely. At this point, it was late in the day, the team was getting burnt out, and I was beginning to fatigue. It was time to call it a day and start fresh the next and final day in the lab.

Day Four

Going into the home stretch, our priority was to perfect the standing performance. The first order at hand, stand with fresh muscles and see if the right leg still kicks out. On the first stand of the day the right leg was still kicking out.

We headed back to the therapy mat for more problem solving. The therapist started to work in order to find the culprit while the engineer programmed the patterns using the Morse Code box. We found that the quad muscles were inducing a slight flexion. We turned back to the data collected from the dynamometer testing. The engineer found the next combination of cuff electrode channels with maximum stimulation and minimum spillover. We tried two different channels; one at full stimulation and the other at 50 percent. We saw some improvement and it was still not the best but it looked good enough to take home and begin using. We then rebalanced the other electrode patterns for a final standing pattern and I was back on the dynamometer machine for more data collection.

We rounded out the final hours going through our checklist: do a balance test, find the final settings for exercise patterns and then the "Stand to Fatigue" test. Here I stood for as long as I could handle or until there was a sign of fatigue, whichever came first. The first stand to fatigue test using the original eight-channel system was about two minutes. With the new system it was 24 minutes, 49 seconds. Quite a difference.

While the engineer returned to his office for the final programming of the take-home patterns, we reflected on the four days with the therapist. There had been a lot of testing. There were new patterns to try at home including the wheelchair propulsion, trunk control, massage, exercise, and standing patterns. My mission was to take the UECU home, use it in the real world, and report back to the research team. We would regroup in the spring to tackle the next phase. There was still a lot to do in the studies. If it was easy, it wouldn't be science.

Christmas came early for me.

Chapter 10: The Rubber Meets the Road

The first stand with the system is not the end point of this research. It simply marks one milestone: the end of the installation/recovery phase of the protocol and the beginning of the rehabilitation and functional use phase. Standing in the lab answers the question, "Is it possible?" but it doesn't answer the question, "How will it be used?"

As a clinical trial participant, this is when the rubber meets the road. This is where my input helps drive the discovery of research. At this point, the research team sent me home with the new standing patterns and the ability to stand using a walker. For the next several months, it would be my job to build standing endurance, improve my comfort level with the system in terms of balance and timing, and push my ability to move around with a swing through gait.

But that is not the only challenge the research team issued. The external control unit is filled with different types of functional use patterns. Patterns for pressure release, trunk control, and wheelchair propulsion to name a few. Over the next few months, I would be challenged to use these patterns in the real world and report back to the research team.

Relieving Pressure in the Air

The first pattern I put to use was on the flight back to Florida after a week in the Cleveland laboratories. Two patterns I used on the plane are aptly named **Glut Shift** and **Glut Shift with Backs**.

For anyone who has flown coach class lately, those seats seem to get smaller and smaller. For a wheelchair user, traveling on the airlines means handing over your only means of mobility. People get upset about taking off their shoes through security. Imagine leaving your only means of getting around in the world on a jet way.

Packed like sardines, there is not a lot of elbow room to spare. This leaves a difficult challenge to be able to lift oneself for a pressure release. Pressure releases are one of the first wheelchair skills taught in rehabilitation. The quick and cheap prevention method is to lift yourself every 15 minutes to relieve pressure. How practical is that? For some who cannot lift themselves, it is not. And for those that can, there are situations, like an airline seat, were it is not possible.

Pressure releases are done to prevent pressure sores or debicutus ulcers, otherwise known as bed sores. According to the Department of Veteran Affairs, one-third of people with spinal cord injuries develop pressure sores. Complications from them kill 60,000 Americans a year—twice the number who die from prostate cancer. One sore can take a person out of daily life for six to 12 months and costs for treatments range from $50,000 to $100,000. It amazes me that our health care system spends more money and effort to treat pressure sores rather than to prevent them. But insurance companies continue to label preventative efforts as "custodial."

For people living with spinal cord injuries, prevention is not custodial—it is a constant battle to protect boney areas such as the butt, spine, and heels. The research team has heard the concern of the paralysis community and they are developing patterns into the system for pressure release using the implanted electrodes.

There is a small team of researchers in Cleveland who are studying pressure points for wheelchair users and discovering ways to use electrical stimulation for prevention. They are affectionately called the "Butt Team." While in Cleveland, we conducted several tests for their data collection. This team is testing different patterns for pressure relief. To conduct the tests, they placed a sensory mat on top of my wheelchair seat cushion and

I transferred on to it. This matt was connected to a computer to gather data.

Using the implanted electrodes, we ran about 12 different series of patterns and watched on the computer screen as the pressure changed. The muscles stimulated with these patterns were very select: the gluteus maximus, lateralis, and the quadreadus. As the electrodes cycled on and off, the computer screen showed areas that change with red (high pressure points) to blue (low pressure points). This work represents one of the most significant and compelling advances for people with spinal cord injuries.

Back in my 18 by 16-inch airline seat, I settled in for a 2 ½ hour flight from Cleveland to Tampa. Pressure lifting every 15 minutes is not possible. But thanks to the research team, I can use **Glut Shift** and **Glut Shift with Backs** for pressure release. For the ride down, I flipped on the external control unit and select **Glut Shift**. This pattern oscillates the right and left butt muscles on and off. If someone was watching me, they could probably see me sway from side to side, but the motion was not enough to disturb the person next to me. This pattern offered me pressure release for my butt but not the spine. The pattern **Glut Shift with Backs** stimulates the butt muscles and the back muscles too. This is perfect for sitting out of my wheelchair on a surface with high back support, like an airline or car seat.

Long periods out of the comfort of my wheelchair seat are prime opportunities for developing pressure sores. These two patterns are a great addition to my prevention arsenal. Where else can I use it? How can I try it in the real world? I posed that question on my social network. So if you see me swaying from side to side with no music playing, you'll know why.

Trunk Control

Looking at wheelchair users, we often focus on the mobility issue. I am often asked the question, "Will you walk again?" But for those with spinal cord injuries, there are so many other hidden issues that can make dramatic impacts on quality of life, such as bladder function, sensation, or spasticity. Don't get me wrong—if I had the opportunity to walk like I did prior to my injury, I'd take it. But in the meantime, there are ways to make my life easier as a wheelchair user.

In this research phase, I was challenged with exploring the functional patterns provided in the implanted standing system. Another one of those patterns is trunk control. The trunk plays a critical role in functional standing. When referring to the trunk, it is the area from the hips to the breast line. These are the muscles often described as the "core" muscle groups.

Trunk stability is a desire among people with spinal cord injuries. According to research published by Dr. Kim Anderson-Erisman, "Targeting Recovery: Priorities of the Spinal Cord-Injured Population," trunk stability is the third highest priority among quadriplegics and paraplegics.

Trunk stability influences how I function in the wheelchair. With my level of spinal cord injury, I am unable to sit without support; I need either a seat back or to hold myself with my arms. With the electrodes turned on, I gain a very straight and effortless sit. Another example is when I reach up for something. I do not have the core muscles to hold myself up. To do so, I use one arm to hold myself and one to reach. Sure, they sell fancy reachers, but anyone who has used one knows that they just don't compare to the use of your own hand.

With the new implanted system, we have added more muscles to the stimulation pattern for trunk control. With the original system, we only stimulated the erector spinae. That gave me some trunk control but it was like sitting on a stilt. If I lost balance, I would fall back in the chair. With the new system, we are now stimulating the erector spinae but also the quadratus lumborum and the gluteus muscles. My posture is straighter and I am much more stable when the system is activated.

Where can I use this? I have been using it for daily activities like folding laundry or washing dishes and also for reaching with more stability. Using the stimulation system is easy and convenient; I just bring my small UECU with me. I am still trying to find more uses for the trunk control function.

Unexpected Benefits

Who doesn't like a good back massage? What if you could get one for free at any time?

In a clinical research trial, investigators can try to predict different outcomes but they truly do not know what will happen until they start working with people, particularly people who can give them feedback. In that valuable feedback, we find unexpected benefits.

While in the Cleveland laboratory, we did several tests on the dynamometer machine. A member of the research team is an engineer dedicated to the exploration of using various channels in the cuff electrodes in order to reduce fatigue. The cuff electrodes are the implanted electrodes that are wrapped around the femoral nerve. Within one implanted electrode are four channels. The challenge is to create the optimum pattern of oscillation of turning the channels on and off to provide muscle stimulation for standing and rest time for the muscle. The goal is to reduce the time for the muscles to fatigue. The dynamometer machine is the main tool for gathering data to get the various experimental patterns.

One morning during my visit to Cleveland in December, we arrived at the laboratory for a two-hour session on the dynamometer machine. The engineer and the principal investigator (PI) were both present. The PI was obviously excited about this research. This was quite evident when he climbed over other equipment to capture the testing activity with his video camera.

After a few tests, the engineer and I established a routine. For one test, we were gathering data for a vibration pattern. He said, "Okay, I am going to turn on your right quad. Ready?"

I responded, "Ready." As we were both looking down at my right thigh muscle, the engineer pressed the start button. Nothing happened. He had a very perplexed look on his face. Then I said, "Well, you obviously did not turn on my right quad, but you did turn on my right back muscle. And it feels really good." The vibrating back muscles felt like a full massage chair.

The muscles that he activated using the vibration pattern are in the lumbar spine area. For anyone who sits for long periods of time, back pain is a common problem. The same issue can apply to wheelchair users. Of course, I inquired about taking this new "Back Massage" home with me. Now, within my repertoire of functional patterns for the implanted system, I have a mobile back massager. What an unexpected benefit!

Test Pattern in the Real World

When an opportunity knocks, it's time to take it.

One of the testing patterns the researchers provided in the external control unit is a wheelchair program. It was created to help propel a manual wheelchair.

The pattern stimulates the gluts, thus providing stability to my hips while I'm in the chair. The pattern also includes stimulation of the erector spinae and the quadradus. This provides trunk control but the stimulation thresholds are lower. This allows enough movement of the shoulders to make wheeling on uneven surfaces easier. Without the stimulation, I would normally wheel a long incline with my torso far forward trying to get the maximum weight forward in the wheelchair.

In my regular daily schedule, I propel mostly short distances. Would I really use a wheelchair propulsion program for this application? No. But there are occasions when I do need to wheel longer distances. While in Miami for the 2011 Olympic Classes Regatta or MOCR, such an opportunity did arise.

The Sunday after racing concluded, the U.S. Sailing Team had a mandatory meeting at the Coconut Grove Sailing Club on the Biscayne Bay waterfront. At the same time, the Miami Marathon was underway, with many road closures in Coconut Grove. Getting to the meeting spot was just not possible with a vehicle so I decided to "hoof it." Tim dropped me off about 10 city blocks away from the meeting spot. It was clearly time to get the morning workout and wheel my way to the waterfront. It was also an opportunity to try the wheelchair propulsion pattern.

Typically when I wheel longer distances, I need to stop periodically to readjust my position in the wheelchair; I might need to sit up straighter, readjust my legs, or straighten my hips. But while using the wheelchair propulsion pattern, this was not necessary. The stimulation kept my body firmly planted in the wheelchair, making distance wheeling much easier. I did have to get used to the stimulation, though, particularly with a bag on my lap, but overall the wheeling required less effort with the stimulation turned on.

As I arrived at the Coconut Grove Sailing Club, the meeting was on the second floor. Absent of any elevator, the only way to get to the second floor is via one of the area's longest ramps. This ramp met ADA codes for gradient but it had six legs doubling back to get you up to the second level. This was hoofing it for sure! My first attempt ascending the ramp was with stimulation. It was no easy task but I tried it and made it up with little hesitation, even with the rubber mat obstacles at the top. It didn't seem like the stimulation was much help.

But later, we went down the ramp for team photos and then needed to ascend back up for the rest of the team meeting. The second attempt ascending the ramp was without stimulation. What a difference. I ascended the ramp much slower this time, causing a back up of other wheelchair users. My arms started to feel the pain since I did not have the stimulation for the trunk muscles to help with the propulsion. Now it was clear that the wheelchair propulsion pattern *did* help when maneuvering up a ramp. Being more erect while wheeling an incline is counter-intuitive from what I had been taught about wheelchair techniques, but it works. I'm sold.

Feeding the Addiction

Spasticity. For those living with spinal cord injury (and other neurological conditions like multiple sclerosis, cerebral palsy and ALS), it is a "secondary" condition that raises its ugly head if not treated. Spasticity comes in many forms. It can come at any time and without warning.

According to the National Institutes of Health, "Spasticity is a condition in which certain muscles are continuously contracted. This contraction causes stiffness or tightness of the muscles and may interfere with movement, speech, and manner of walking. Spasticity is usually caused by damage to the portion of the brain or spinal cord that controls voluntary movement. Symptoms may include hypertonicity (increased muscle tone), clonus (a series of rapid muscle contractions), exaggerated deep tendon reflexes, muscle spasms, scissoring (involuntary crossing of the legs), and fixed joints. The degree of spasticity varies from mild muscle stiffness to severe, painful, and uncontrollable muscle spasms."

When I was first injured, I had a doctor explain to me that I would develop uncontrollable muscle spasms that I would have to manage on a regular basis. She wasn't kidding. Within a few months, I developed the muscle spasms as she described. At times, they were so bad that a spasm would throw me out of my wheelchair.

There are ways to manage spasticity. At first, I tried the common way, pharmaceuticals. Basically, these are muscle-relaxing drugs, but I found that I couldn't function mentally while taking those drugs so I stopped. There are other ways to manage spasticity; standing, electrical stimulation, yoga, and stretching; which leads me to how the new implanted system helps me to manage spasticity.

There are two ways that I have been using the implanted system to manage spasticity. Standing with the system is the obvious way. The more I stand using electrical stimulation, the more my muscle spasms relax. Tim and I went canoeing for a two-day excursion in southwest Florida. Figuring we had enough equipment to bring with us, I opted to leave the walker behind and not stand for two days. Within 24 hours, the spasms started to come back. Within 48 hours, my body was craving a stand. I had to feed the addiction.

The other way to manage spasticity is by using the pattern called **Extends All**. This pattern is an exercise function that turns all the implanted electrodes on for 15 seconds and then off for 10 seconds. The pattern duration is an hour. This pattern was originally created to build the endurance fibers in the implanted muscle groups. But more important, I found it really helps me manage spasticity. It relaxes my muscles so the spasms don't awaken me in the middle of the night.

Some say that managing spasticity using electrical stimulation is a double-edged sword. On one hand, electrical stimulation relaxes the frequency of the muscle spasms, but on the other hand, the spasms that do occur are stronger. I can attest that this statement is true, at least for my case.

Using electrical stimulation is not a quick fix either. IFESS (the International Functional Electrical Stimulation Society) warns that the maximum benefit of using electrical stimulation to manage spasticity "may not be realized until it has been used for one to two hours per day for one to three months."

For me, keeping a daily exercise regime to manage a few occasional spasms is a viable solution. With that in mind, I continue to feed my addiction to electrical stimulation and keep the spasticity monster at bay.

Going the Distance

Okay, using the new implanted system, I'm able to stand with a walker. But I was able to stand with a walker using the original implanted system. So what's all the hype about? On the surface, it appears to be functionally the same. In reality, the new implanted system provides those small upgrades that make a big difference, almost like going from a 3G cellular network to 4G.

However, as with any phase of this research process, results are not immediate. When I first stood with the new implanted system, the endurance test for standing duration was a maximum of 24 minutes. That is pretty good, but there is more.

One of the goals of this new upgraded system is to allow me to stand and move around short distances using crutches. Several years ago, I tried to use crutches with the original system. It was possible but very difficult. I never became independent with crutches and it was never functional for me to stand with the crutches. I went back to using the system with a walker and being able to functionally stand and move around.

At this point with the new system, I was back to that base level and using a walker. On my next visit to the lab in Cleveland, we would begin working with the physical therapist to start the process of using crutches. Again, change is never instant.

How did I prepare for this next lab session in March? As a research participant, it is my responsibility to be prepared for each phase of the project. To prepare, I worked on increasing the daily standing time. Did I cheat? Well, yes. I had days when I only stood for five to 10 minutes. For the most part, though, I stood for 30 to 40 minutes per day.

Endurance for standing is not the only skill I needed to build. The other was getting balanced and comfortable with the new standing system. For building that skill, I started doing laps. With my swing through gait, I lift the walker, move it forward, then lift both legs to swing the body forward. When I lift the walker, I am gaining the confidence and comfort of being balanced with the standing system alone providing support. The motion also builds my upper body strength and endurance. These are the same muscles I would need when we started working with crutches.

Slowly increasing the distance I moved helped me prepare for the testing time in the lab. Committing to daily exercise and skill building helped me achieve better results in the lab.

I had just returned from a U.S. Sailing Team training camp in Miami. While staying in my teammate's condo in Coconut Grove, I did some laps in the courtyard. The beauty of this implanted system is that regardless of where I may be, I can still bring the system with me. I can keep training to go the distance. Plus, I could continue preparing for our sacred lab time in March.

Beta Testing

Have you ever tested a beta version of new software? It may be a new feature on Google or new software developed by Microsoft, Oracle, or Intuit. The purpose of testing beta versions is to find the bugs in systems prior to it being released as a final version. It is a way of finding technical challenges. These challenges just cannot be anticipated by engineering design but they surface as the technology is handed over to the user community. My implanted stimulation system is no different.

There have been some anatomic challenges particularly when it came to the surgical implantation. Now, as I used the system in the real world other technical challenges started to surface. Regardless, this is the reason for a clinical trial; it is a way to test the beta version.

One technical issue surfaced while using the system that relates to the coupling of the coil to the implanted receiver. The receiver is fully implanted into my abdominal area. The external components consist of a coil and a universal external control unit. To activate the system, the coil is taped to the skin directly over the implanted receiver; the coil is connected to the UECU. The UECU sends messages through the coil to the implanted receiver to activate the implanted electrodes. Getting a good connection between the receiver and the coil is called coupling.

Much like being in a wifi hotspot, the signal between the coil and the receiver can be strong with a good placement or weak if not placed properly. The coils are available in two lengths, a short form of about 24 inches or a long form; which is 72 inches. With the new IST-16 implanted receiver, we discovered that the coupling of the coils is different between the short and the long versions. If the long coil is placed properly over the implanted receiver, then the signal is strong and consistent. However, if the short coil is placed in the same location at the same power level, then the coupling fades in and out and there is not a strong signal between the implanted receiver and the UECU. When the signal fades, the electrodes deactivate. This is not so good when I'm depending on those electrodes to stand. Fortunately for me, we discovered this issue when I was using the system for leg lift exercises.

During my last visit to the Cleveland laboratory, we spent at least two hours trying to determine the appropriate power output settings to optimize the coupling. The solution was to control power output to the two systems independently and increase power output to the new system. We agreed that I would try it at the new setting, give feedback, and the engineer could make more adjustments as needed. At this point, my original system was set at one-half power and the new system is set at three-fourths power, so there is still room to increase if necessary.

The tradeoff that comes with higher power output is a quicker drain on the battery. This means that I have less usage time before the battery needs a recharge. That is one variable that I did not take into account. While using the UECU, there is a safety feature for the low battery. If the battery runs low, a **Low Bat** visual cue appears on the UECU along with a high-pitch warning sound. Typically there is a use time of at least six minutes until the battery is completely out of power. I was still getting comfortable with the shorter battery life as the UECU began reaching the alarm state more quickly, so I had to be aware of that when I'm using the system for functional activities.

These technical challenges don't have a quick and easy solution. As each issue is discovered, the feedback was sent to the technical team, who would troubleshoot the problem for a potential permanent resolution. This is the process of effective technical design. I'm sure devices like the Android and the iPad were not perfect the first time out of the design lab. As with most new technologies, it takes people using devices to discover the deficiencies and build an overall better system.

Chapter 11: Preparing for Paralympics

Once per year, the U.S. Sailing Team Paralympic members trek to Birmingham, AL and the Lakeshore Foundation campus. There are 18 team members with a variety of disabilities: amputees, stroke, spinal cord injury, and visual impairments. It is a time that the team gathers together to check in with our fitness, physical training, nutrition, psychology, and logistical programs for the sport of sailboat racing.

Lakeshore Foundation is one of the national training centers for Paralympic sports. Name a Paralympic summer sport and more than likely, it is represented at this facility; quad rugby, swimming, goalball, wheelchair basketball—you get the point.

When we arrived at the Birmingham airport, a big wheelchair-accessible van was there for curbside pick up. Piling into the van, we headed over to the Lakeshore property and proceeded up the winding path between buildings, dormitories, and rehabilitation facilities to the top of the hill where the main training facility and athlete dormitory is located.

The four-day visit is filled with activities from 8 am through 9 pm. The focus for the U.S. Sailing Team this year is fitness and communication. On the fitness side, we reviewed our exercise plans and met with the therapist to go over exercises that will best prepare us for the roles we have on the sailboat. My teammate, JP, and I took the time to meet with one of the trainers.

We also went through a battery of tests to benchmark our progress year over year. There are a variety of tests for speed, endurance, coordination, and strength. This was also a good time to see if some of the stimulation patterns have an influence on the performance of these tests. Two tests in particular were prime ground for trying the implanted stimulation system to see if they influence outcomes.

One test is strictly for measuring endurance. It is the 12-minute run/walk/wheel. On the track in the main gymnasium, we have a starting line and wheel around the track as fast as we can for 12 minutes. Now, 12 minutes does not seem like a long time, but try wheeling at full speed for that long and just one minute seems longer than you ever thought. In previous years, I ran this test without any stimulation and completed about 3960 ft. in the allotted time. This year, I performed that same task using the wheelchair propulsion pattern programmed into the UECU. The results in 12 minutes I wheeled 4097 ft. There does not seem to be a big difference between the two. However, there is one caveat. In previous years, I was using pneumatic tires and this year, I switched to solid tires, which add more friction. The conclusion: we need more tests on the wheelchair propulsion pattern to see if there is a definite benefit or not.

The other test of the stimulation patterns in action is the Trim Test. Designed specifically for sailors, this is a test of pulling on 45½ ft of line with 25 lbs attached to the end and thera-band on the end to add resistance. During the test, we pull on the line as fast as we can until we reach the end of the line. The observers measure the number of pulls and the time to complete the task. This is a measure of speed, coordination, and upper body and core muscle strength. It is a prime test for the trunk stimulation pattern. The trunk pattern stimulates the four electrodes in the back (two on the erector spinae and two on the quadradus) plus the gluteus maximus muscles. The pattern provides good posture and core muscle support. At Lakeshore, we tried several different tests with different resistance levels and with and without stimulation. After several consecutive tests, we did not

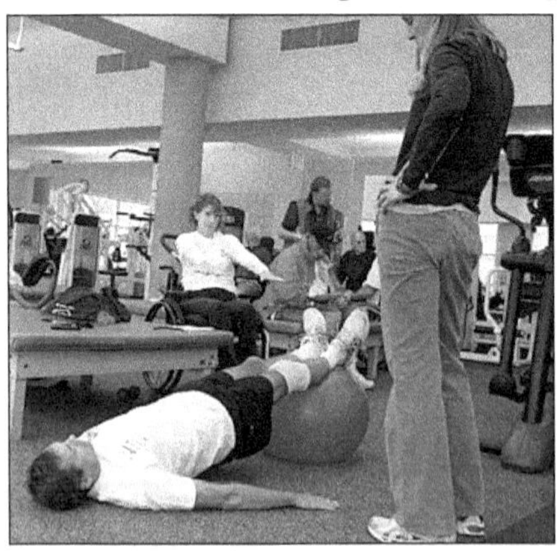

JP and I work out at the Lakeshore facility.

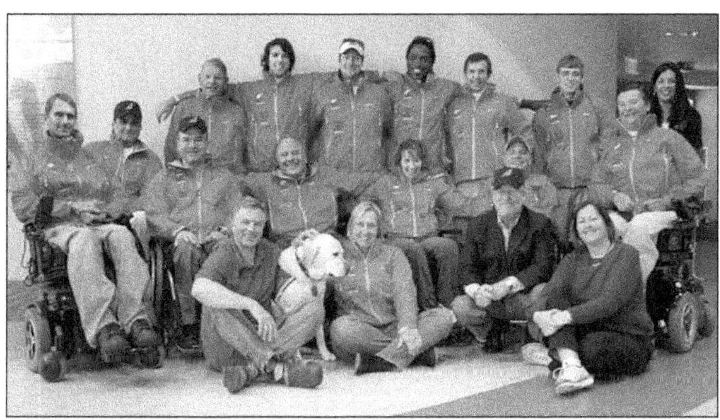

U.S. Sailing Team photo from Lakeshore (Photo courtesy U.S. Sailing)

find a significant performance difference in the outcomes. However, the big difference was the observation by three team support staff. They all commented on how the stimulation provided a noticeably better posture and the mechanics of the movement was dramatically improved. Recommendations from the coach: practice more with the stimulation.

Even though we did not see the dramatic breakthrough in the performance data of the stimulation patterns, this was a good time to benchmark and see how it applied in the real world. Each test was only performed once. As any researcher knows, repetition will uncover the true data.

As we left the hill for the end of the weekend, we did have a great time improving our fitness potential and communication within and outside of the team. We even had some fun team-building exercises like synchronized swimming and wheelchair flag football. Yes, I can be a linebacker in a wheelchair.

Chapter 12: Life as a Lab Rat

It comes with the territory. Being a participant in clinical research includes being involved with various laboratory experiments; some are simple and others not so much. They are all in the interest of developing a viable device. Over the five-day visit in March 2011 to the Cleveland FES laboratory, we conducted an array of experiments with the standing system. Some related directly to standing performance but others are testing additional functional patterns of the system such as pressure relief, wheelchair propulsion, and trunk control. This is an overview of the experiments from a participant's perspective.

A unique feature of the upgraded system is the cuff electrodes hugging my femoral nerve controlling the group of muscles in the upper thigh area. One engineer is focusing on how most effectively to design and execute an oscillation pattern for the quadriceps to decrease fatigue and gain optimum performance while standing. For this visit, we had several sessions together on the dynamometer. The engineer focused solely on the right leg. Along the way, each new stimulation pattern adopted a new nickname like "sinusoid," "carousel," and "vibration." Most mornings, I would have coffee and dynamometer. We would not see the final results in this visit but it was a key step to getting to longer standing times.

Speaking of fatigue, we ran several stand-to-fatigue (STF) tests to determine my maximal standing times. With four different configurations, each day we would conduct one STF test. For each test, we would place our bets on standing duration. I would stand with the given configuration until I couldn't handle it or a muscle showed signs of fatigue, which is typically the bending of the knee or more pressure on my arms while standing. The configurations and standing times were:

- Standing with the original hips and trunk electrodes (Glut max, hamstring and erector spinae) and the original epimysial electrodes on the quads. Time: 3 min 40 sec.

- Standing with all hips and trunk electrodes (Glut max, hamstring, glut med, post adductors, quadradus and erector spinae) and the original epimysial electrodes on the quads. Time: 4 min 7 sec.

- Standing with the original hips and trunk electrodes (Glut max, hamstring and erector spinae) and the new cuff electrodes on the quads. Time: 34 min.

- Standing with all hips and trunk electrodes (Glut max, hamstring, glut med, post adductors, quadratus and erector spinae) and the new cuff electrodes on the quads. Time: 50 min 4 sec.

These STF times not only show the value of the new cuff electrodes but also the other new electrodes in my hips and trunk.

Another area of experimentation was to develop a stimulation pattern to reduce pressure in the seated position. As I explained earlier, pressure sores are a constant threat to people living with spinal cord injuries. If stimulation can help prevent a pressure sore, it can provide great benefit not only to the person using the wheelchair but also the entire healthcare system.

On this visit the engineers tested three different pressure-relief patterns to find out which would be most effective. For each variation, they would gather data on the oxygen in my skin using sensors taped to my rear end and the pressure on my seat using a sensor mat on my wheelchair cushion. For each pattern, they would activate the stimulation for five minutes and then have me sit quietly for five minutes. I think the sitting quietly was more of a challenge for me than for the researchers. Once the data were analyzed, they used it to create the most useful pressure relief pattern, then returned to test that pattern against conventional pressure relief methods, such as lifting every 15 minutes or reclining in the wheelchair.

Two of the days in the Cleveland laboratory were dedicated to analyzing the effects of stimulation on wheelchair propulsion and trunk stability. Most of these experiments were conducted with specialized equipment housed at the Louis Stokes Veterans Administration Hospital in Cleveland and with the Principal Investigator pacing in the background.

My homework assignment before traveling up to Cleveland for this visit was to test the wheelchair propulsion pattern in the real world. As I did, my biggest complaint was the fact that the stimulation would forcibly rotate my knees and anything that I was carrying on my lap would fall off. Realistically, I would not use the wheelchair propulsion pattern for short distances, but for longer treks in the wheelchair. And in that situation, I would most likely be carrying something on my lap. Plus, when I wheeled on uneven surfaces my knees would still wobble around.

With this feedback, the therapist and engineer worked together to try to find a viable solution. They adjusted the stimulation pattern to hold my knees together but for my left side it was not so simple. To help solve this problem, we adjusted the stimulation between the left glut max and the left post adductor. The engineer would adjust the stimulation pattern, turn on the system, and we would then observe which muscle would win the battle. If the glut max won, then the knee would rotate out. If the post adductor won, then the knee would rotate in. During these tests, my knee was flipping in and out—entertaining everyone in the room. In the end, we finally found just the right balance between the two muscle groups for a more functional wheelchair propulsion pattern.

Now that we had the pattern established, it was time to collect data. The general goal is to stimulate targeted hip and trunk muscles for a more rigid seated position while minimizing the energy lost due to the body wobbling in the wheelchair and improving the efficiency of pushing. A specialized wheel was placed onto my wheelchair to measure how hard I pushed and in which direction. Unfortunately, the wheel didn't start up the first day and the team couldn't get it working. After digging into the guts of the wheel, they were able to get it operating properly but this backed up all the experiments into the next day.

There were two basic experiments for the wheelchair propulsion pattern. The first tested the pattern while wheeling on ramps. The team set up a room with two ramps; one at 10 degrees of slope and the other at 5 degrees of slope. Each ramp length was about 6 feet. For the experiment, on cue I would wheel up one of the ramps either with stimulation or without stimulation. The research team would measure the time to wheel up the ramp, the number of pushes I needed, plus the data collected from the wheel. After several trials, there was no real observable difference with and without using stimulation.

Feedback from this experiment is that the real value of the wheelchair propulsion pattern seems to be for long distances. But how can we evaluate its value for longer distances? This is where participants can influence research. I led them to the ultimate test-bed for a ramp with distance, slope, and resistance. At the Louis Stokes VA hospital, there is a very long incline with various slopes from the parking garage to the main hospital. Plus, this long incline is carpeted, making it more difficult to propel a wheelchair. Off we go to the incline, which is the main

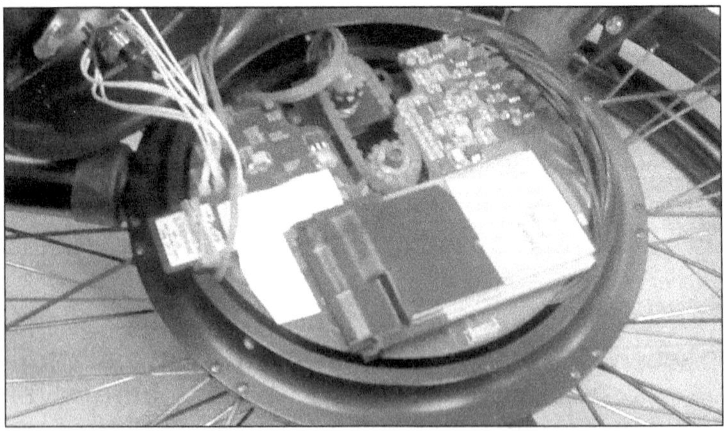

The researchers used a "smart" wheel on my wheelchair to collect data.

route between the parking garage and the hospital. We attempted to run the experiments while keeping the normal traffic from interfering, so the general hospital patrons must have thought we were crazy. But in the end, it worked. We tested the incline with and without stimulation and observed that the duration and intensity of the pushes were reduced with stimulation. I suspected testing like this will surface again on my next visit.

The other experiment involved using a motion-capture system in the Gait Laboratory. This camera system is the same one used by the motion picture industry to develop animation and computer-generated special effects. But for this application, the research team used the system to analyze movement while propelling a wheelchair with and without stimulation. They placed small reflective balls on key areas of my body such as the shoulder, hips, and elbows. When I was in the viewing area of the cameras, I could wave my arms like a ghost and a "connect the dots" image of the reflective balls would move in real-time on the computer screen. The stresses and strains on my shoulder could be computed from the positions of my arms and trunk, together with the data from the wheels. The question is whether stimulation affects both how I push the wheelchair and ultimately the wear and tear on my shoulders.

The experiment was conducted by having me propel the wheelchair at a constant speed across the floor of the laboratory; some trials with stimulation and some without stimulation. Two engineers had the computer systems connected to the cameras and we had my mom on the video camera. One engineer would call "Ready," and the other "Set," Then my mom would call "Go." We repeated this sequence a total of 20 times. The two videos below show the experiments with and without stimulation. It is difficult to tell the difference by eye, but focus on my posture in the wheelchair.

The final set of experiments explored the effects of stimulation on my trunk stability. The first experiment was a rowing test. A bar was attached to the dynamometer to simulate a rowing exercise machine. The dynamometer kept the tension and speed of movement at a constant rate and the researchers would measure the force I exerted as I pulled the bar toward me. This movement would be done with and without stimulation 10 times each. From personal observation, without stimulation I would arch my back and strain my lower back. With stimulation, the movement was much easier with a straight posture.

The second trunk stability test gathered data about my ability to extend my hips and back to press into an upright position. The test was conducted in three different angles of the trunk; upright, 15 degrees bent forward, and 30 degrees bent forward. For each angle position, they would test the baseline (me not moving), pushing back with no stimulation, pushing back only using stimulation, and pushing back with both my effort and stimulation. The pushing back would be for five seconds followed by 25 seconds of rest. The engineer kept time, monitored the computer screens, and attempted to keep me on track.

As we progressed through this experiment, the upright position was not that bad. But as we moved to the 15 degrees and the 30 degrees, it became progressively more difficult. At some point, my face was completely red and I needed to take a break. What we will do for research. The saving grace during this test was the little image on the computer screen.

Although the system is called the Standing System, there are many other applications that can be derived from the various implanted electrodes. These experimental patterns need to be proven with data and analysis. As users, we can provide feedback of the impact, potential uses in the real world and provide observations. In the end, medical research needs data to prove comparative effectiveness before it can be a viable option in the health system. With that in mind, these experiments are a necessity to allow people to get access to the technology.

Transition to Crutches

The ability to stand with crutches was one of the original goals and reasons for getting the upgraded standing system. I have been standing with the eight-channel implanted system for 12 years. This new goal is a lofty one for a quadriplegic.

The first crutch-standing attempts took place over the five-day March 2011 stretch in the lab. We squeezed in training with the crutches around various other experiments that required special equipment, the scheduling of other researchers, and alternative lab time.

After three months of standing with the upgraded standing system, it was time to set the walker aside and begin standing with the crutches. The transition was not easy. Just like taking the training wheels off a bike, converting to crutches is an odd feeling at first. While preparing to stand, I no longer have the comfort of a walker as a security box around me and I need to trust the implanted system.

The first day in the lab, it was time to put the new standing system to the test. To make the transition easier, I transferred to a lab mat and the therapist raised the level up to help make the sit-to-stand transition easier. The first attempts would be with gaiter-aid crutches; these are Canadian crutches with a four-prong foot base. With two spotters (one being the therapist), I activated the system. *One, two, three, and up.* But I needed help and lots of it. Using the gaiter-aids proved to be more difficult than expected. We tried a few more standing attempts, but no success.

The therapist observed that the gaiter-aids may not be the right tool. She took the crutches and maneuvered herself around the lab using the gaiter-aids. Not impressed by the stability of the gaiter-aides, the therapist went back into the equipment closet and returned with a set of Lofstrand crutches with a standard single point base. "Let's try these." With a few more standing attempts, there was some improvement. But it still was not a smooth stand, as with a walker. In the typical research team fashion, we began to troubleshoot and dissect the problem to find solutions.

One issue is my ability to activate the system. For years, I have been able to take my hand off the walker to press the buttons on the UECU to activate and deactivate the system. With crutches, it is much more difficult to press the button and hold onto the crutches at the same time. There was a technical solution for this, however. The engineer stepped out of the lab to his locker of equipment and returned with a finger switch. This is a long coil that connects to the UECU. On the end of the coil is a ring to wear on my finger. Attached to this ring is a control panel of smaller buttons for the UECU. I can wear the ring and activate the system with my finger while keeping my hands on the crutches. To properly accommodate me, the engineer turned into a jeweler and fit me properly with the optimum ring size and then adjusted the finger switch to fit me.

The most compelling discovery we made was that standing with the crutches reveals the discrepancies in the system. These discrepancies do not surface nor are they easy to compensate for when using a walker. In other words, while using a walker I can easily "suck it up," and move around despite suboptimal stimulation. But standing with crutches, "sucking it up" is not so easy. In the end, this became an engineering challenge to tweak the system to get to that perfect stand.

What did we discover? For quite some time, when using a walker and using a swing-through gait, my right leg would kick forward. While trying to solve this problem, we focused on muscles on the right side of the body. We adjusted about every electrode to try to find the culprit with no success. While working with crutches, the therapist observed that my left hip was rotating back and this was an epiphany toward finding a solution. The culprit was not a muscle on the right side, but it was my left gluteus maximus muscle. This muscle was contracting and rotating my left hip back and in turn swinging my right leg forward. We gave the box to the engineer to program the UECU to lower the left glut muscle. Problem solved.

The right leg issue was not the only discrepancy that surfaced while using the crutches. Transitioning from sit to stand was not a smooth movement. We had several sit-to-stand practices, and I needed a double rock of the upper body to get enough momentum to stand up; I called this the "double oomph" maneuver. The engineer offered a little technical help with this too. He programmed into the UECU a booster shot for the stand. This gave me a stronger muscle contraction during the sit-to-stand transition. Technically, what he programmed was an increase in frequency to 30 hertz for 10 seconds and then a decrease to 20 hertz for the remainder of the stand. Using this booster shot, I put the "double oomph" to rest and then I could just concentrate on one good transition from sit to stand.

The troubleshooting was not over yet. With the booster shot, my left foot would rotate outward. When I stood with the walker, this did not happen. But while standing with the crutches, the problem would surface. We took the team back to the lab mat to troubleshoot and to find the muscle that was the culprit of this undesired movement. It ended up being the left hamstring. After many trials and adjustments to the pulse width for this muscle, we found a good setting to allow a stable stand and eliminate the left foot rotation.

On a Friday afternoon near the end of the day, we did the final round of standing. In position at the edge of the lab mat and with the crutches in place, I clicked the go button to stand. *One, two, three, stand.* Success! We achieved a smooth transition from sit to stand, although with some quirky muscle recruitment. "Okay, let's sit and do that again to make sure it wasn't a mistake or a fluke." I rested for 20 seconds, then got into position. "Everyone ready? Go." *One, two, three, stand.* Again, success. The therapist then lowered the mat to the same level as my wheelchair. Let's try it again. It worked.

Were the stands perfect at this point? No. Was I independent using them? No. So, I chose to leave the crutches in the lab while I returned to Florida. In a short time, I would travel back to the lab for more training and experiments. We hadn't met the goal yet, but we made great progress in five days. With some further investment of blood, sweat, and tears we should be on track to achieving our goal.

Up for the Count

One, ha ha ha. Two, ha ha ha. Three, ha ha ha. Four, ha ha ha.

Taking inspiration from our purple friend from Sesame Street, Count von Count, the April 2011 visit to the Cleveland lab focused on learning how to count to four.

Actually, the goal was to stand up out of my own wheelchair

and to do so unassisted, otherwise labeled by the therapists as "hands free standing." Timing is everything to achieve this goal. If the count is late, my legs and hips activate before my upper body is ready. If the count is early, then the first part of getting up is completely reliant on my arm strength. For years, I've been standing with the walker and I've gotten lazy with the timing. Nearly nine years ago, Alan Alda interviewed me for an episode of Scientific American Frontiers. While relatively new to standing in that episode, I had remarked about the critical nature of counting to three. The Count surfaces again.

The emphasis was on training for standing. To start off, we did a little more tweaking. This time the engineer decreased the stimulation ramp-up time from 3 seconds to 1 second. This seemed to help with the sit-to-stand from the therapy mat at both a high level and at the level of my wheelchair height. So, the next move was to stand out of my wheelchair. But we had some situational challenges.

Achieving a good stand is reliant on getting your shoulders over your knees and your foot position under you. With my rigid wheelchair, the footplate is the obstacle for proper foot placement. After a little inspection, we found that the footplate was not welded to the frame of the wheelchair, but instead was a removable component. We broke out the tools and Voila! Proper foot placement.

Sit-to-stand should be perfect now, right? Not so fast. With the change in the ramp time down to 1 second and the need to learn how to count, the difference in ramping time triggered a flexion spasm in my hip. When I tried to stand from the wheelchair, my hips flexed and I was unable to straighten my torso. The therapists called this my "old lady stand." What we found is that this spasm went away after the muscle is stimulated for a little while. Our tweaking solution: create a "warm up" pattern to stimulate the muscle while still seated and to work out the spasm.

Since all of the electrodes arc implanted above the knee, I do not have any muscle movement or contractions to stabilize the calf, ankle, or foot. Because of this, I need to wear an ankle

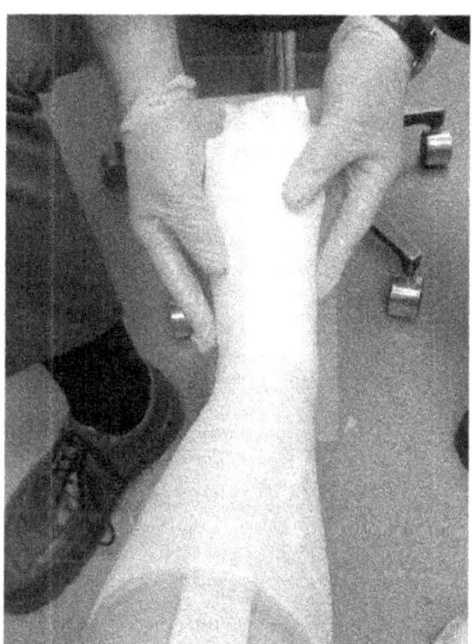

Getting fitted for new AFO

foot orthosis (AFO). This is a brace made out of molded plastic and Velcro that fits into a shoe. The pair that I have been using was 12 years old. The Velcro had been replaced several times and they had been exposed to their share of sunscreen and salt water. It was time to get fitted for a new pair and we had an appointment to meet the prosthesist. He took the old pair and put them on the counter. Over the years, AFOs have changed form and the bottom of the brace does not lie flat on the ground. It was definitely time for new ones.

The process of getting fitted is much like getting a cast for a broken bone. The prosthesist marks the skin for pressure points and slips on a sock-like material over the calf and foot. He then wets a roll of fiberglass and rolls it around the material. (Yes, I asked. It is not the same fiberglass to fix a boat) After taking a short while for the fiberglass to set, he then cuts the cast off. He will use the cast to mold a new set of AFOs and they should be ready for my next visit.

With the tweaking done and appointments completed, it was back to the lab to get down to business, learning how to count. I started standing out of the wheelchair but it was not as easy as it seemed. The placement of the crutches has a big influence on success. We tried many placement options: crutches far forward or far back, crutches in close or out far. It took many trials to find the right placement. If they were too far forward, I didn't have the leverage to push up. If they were too far back, my torso fell forward on the sit-to-stand process. Reminiscent of Goldilocks, we finally found the position that was "just right."

Now, it all boiled down to practice. In one day, we would do 20 to 40 sit-to-stands. Doesn't seem like much? Just try it. Stand out of a chair 20 times in a row. You will feel it. But with practice came skill. The number of bad stands started to fade and the good stands started to dominate.

After four days of practice, the last day in the lab was the final exam to see if I was independent enough to take the crutches home with me. To pass the final exam, I had to impress the therapist and prove with confidence that I could be safe using the crutches. It was all about hands-free standing. This is where the therapists are hovering but they provide no assistance while I use the system to stand. After several practice stands, I was ready for hands-free standing. With a crowd forming, I choked. During the final exam, the bad stands won.

In the end, I was released to bring the crutches home with me for the next month to practice with restrictions. I would only use the crutches to practice sit to stand and I could only use the crutches if I had Tim monitoring me. Yes! I may have choked the exam, but in the end we made big strides on this visit and I would be going home with the crutches. To make sure that I complied with these restrictions, my mom packaged up the crutches so I could not use them before Tim got home.

But let's get to the real reason I traveled up to the Cleveland lab, and that was to learn how to count. Just like practicing a dance routine, counting is everything. *One, two, three four, one two, three, four.* But as the routine became second nature, the counting faded and the moves became more natural. Learning how to stand using crutches is a skill to be refined only through proper technique and practice.

Alternative Patterns

Aside from all the stand training conducted during the April visit to the lab, the researchers stayed true to form including several lab experiments. Here is a review of the various experiments and what we discovered.

Again, each morning I spent 30 to 60 minutes on the dynamometer for testing of the cuff electrodes around the femoral nerve to control the quad muscle group. This is all still data collection.

We also did some testing of the patterns for trunk stability, and particularly the wheelchair propulsion pattern. This pattern stimulates the quadratus, erector spinae, gluteus max, and the post adductors. Again, I got my workout but this time I pulled in the research team with me. This experiment entailed six-minute tests of propelling the wheelchair around a course. Previously, we conducted this experiment in the patient ward of the VA hospital. The patient ward proved to be crowded with unpredictable obstacles. This time, we moved the course to a construction area of the hospital, so our only obstacles were the construction workers (and we did almost run a few of them over). For each six-minute experiment, I propelled my wheelchair with one member of the research team running ahead of me to keep the track clear while two members ran behind me. During each experiment, my mom remained seated and counted the laps while the Smart Wheel on my chair collected data.

Between each experiment, we were allotted a five-minute break. During one of our breaks, a supervisor from the construction team introduced himself and asked, "So, what are you guys doing here?" Before any member of the research team could respond, I chimed in with, "Oh, we're conducting an obesity study and we have these subjects run around a course to see their progress." The therapist spoke up while pointing at a tall, thin engineer, "Yeah, he's lost at least 300 lbs." We had the supervisor believing us for a moment but then we broke down and told him about the wheelchair propulsion testing.

Discovering new ways to use the programmable patterns is a staple of this research program. As one of the experiments, we attempted to see if the trunk or the wheelchair propulsion stimulation patterns might aid transfers in and out of the wheelchair. We started by transferring onto a therapy mat at a high height (much like the height of hotel beds these days). I attempted it without stimulation and had a difficult time with the transfer.

We then tried the same transfer using the trunk stability pattern, but it proved to be more difficult. Finally, we attempted the transfer again while using the wheelchair propulsion pattern. This time, it proved to be helpful.

I wasn't sold yet. So, we increased the height of the mat and tried the experiments again. The wheelchair propulsion pattern again proved to be most beneficial.

The true test is taking the patterns out into the real world. For this visit, I stayed in Cleveland over a weekend and was staying in a hotel nestled in a business park that was nearly abandoned over the weekend. Still not sold on the wheelchair propulsion pattern helping with transfers, I attempted several times to transfer in and out of the hotel bed, which was a typical very high bed. On the previous nights, I had to struggle to transfer into the bed each evening. This time, I attempted the daily routine using the stimulation. It succeeded at converting a difficult task into a piece of cake.

Still trying to understand the value of the wheelchair propulsion pattern, I took advantage of the abandoned parking garage. Starting on the ground level, I wheeled progressively up the floors of the parking garage. For each floor, I would attempt one with stimulation and one without stimulation until I reached the top. For me, the long inclines were much easier using the wheelchair propulsion programs. I was not progressing faster, but the effort that I needed to exert was greatly reduced, particularly the stress on my shoulders, and I could wheel up the long incline without taking a break.

Now that I've proven to myself that the pattern is valuable, we will see how I can integrate the pattern into everyday life.

Arm Wrestling Match

We had progressed along enough in this research to get down to three main testing areas: cuff electrodes, trunk stability, and standing training with crutches. In the name of research, the team typically designs experiments and recruits participants, like me, to work through the experimental process. As a participant, I give them my feedback during the experiments and also try to relate the application to the real world.

This lab visit in May 2011 was no different. The first day in Cleveland, I was back on the dynamometer for more testing of the cuff electrodes. In fact, every morning was dedicated to testing of various oscillation patterns. The data gathered here would help determine the most efficient pattern uses of the four-channel cuff electrodes implanted around the femoral nerve. For most of the week, each morning was focused on fatigue testing, which includes stimulation of the quadriceps for a duration of 30 minutes for each leg. With fatigue testing, we needed a rest period to allow the muscles to recover. We all have our morning routines. Some of us like to exercise, others read the paper, but my routine had become coffee on the dynamometer.

Aside from this routine, there were also more sporadic experiments. Each lab visit was greeted with an unexpected barrage of experiments. Trunk stability was a hot topic. One afternoon was dedicated to testing the trunk stability in the FES Motion Laboratory at the Louis Stokes VA hospital. Away in the basement of the hospital is a lab dedicated to motion testing. One engineer is the expert with the camera data gathering motion system. This system is similar to that used in motion picture production, particularly for animation.

For this experiment, they placed a therapy mat in the middle of the room and to one side were three strings of beads with reflective balls hanging at calculated intervals. To set up my body, the research team mounted reflective balls on several of my upper body joints, on my sternum, and back of the neck, on each side of the hip, and on my forehead and an extended tail on, well, my tailbone. The movement of the reflector balls was captured by the cameras, transmitted to the computer system, and recorded as data points.

For this experiment, I perched on the edge of the therapy mat facing the ceiling strings. At random, I was instructed to perform a reaching movement; some with an empty box, some with a box of rocks, some with stimulation, and some without stimulation. The research therapist was seated adjacent to me on the official therapist square rolling stool. She was there monitoring my movements. For some of the reaching experiments, she really needed to do the limbo to get out of my way. In these experiments, the research team attempted to find how trunk stability stimulation impacts reaching ability. The video of reaching without stimulation compared to with stimulation is pretty compelling. But in this experiment, we noticed that with stimulation, I was able to reach further but was fishing to the stability point.

At the time, the system was delivering stimulation to the erector spinae, quadradus and the gluteus maximus. The contraction of the gluts were rotating my knees. After one set of experiments, we changed the trunk stability pattern to include the above muscle groups plus the post adductors. This brought the knees together. A small change to the stimulation pattern dramatically changed my reaching ability and trunk stability.

After this change to the pattern, we continued with the remaining tests and I kept the new trunk stability pattern for real world use.

Speaking of real world uses, the FES laboratory does not always offer true real world applications. But on occasion, it can. One morning after spending my allotted two hours on the dynamometer, we were hanging out in the lab while allowing my quadriceps to rest before beginning stand training. The topic of arm wrestling came up and as it turns out a member of the research team is quite the arm wrestler. She, yes she, is a retired nurse working for several research programs. Apparently, she has been unbeatable with the FES Center team for those brave enough to arm wrestle her.

In the name of research, we decided to test the trunk stability stimulation pattern in a real world application. She was to arm wrestle me while I used the trunk stability stimulation. Yes, we had a nurse arm wrestling a quadriplegic, but it was in the name of research. We tried one trial without stimulation and she beat me. Then, I turned on the stimulation to my trunk pattern electrodes and wrestled again. Did I win? Well, no, but I put up a good fight.

You can watch the arm wrestling at:

http://www.youtube.com/watch?v=ZiSKdzTqENY

It is amazing what we will do for research. Sometimes, it can be really boring but on other occasions the experiments can be quite entertaining. In the end, it is all in the name of research.

The Post Adductors

Who would think of the post adductor (PA) muscles as a significant muscle group? Over the previous several months, I had been focusing on the quadriceps, the gluts, or the quadradus. But the post adductors? They are nice to have but how much do they really help? They always seemed to me as a nice addition for balance but I could live without them, right? No way! Apparent during the May visit to the Cleveland FES Center laboratory, the PA plays an important role in so many of the stimulation patterns. (For the anatomically challenged, PA are the muscles on the inside of the thigh)

To be true, they surfaced during my visit in April with the wheelchair propulsion pattern. My biggest complaint about the original stimulation pattern for wheelchair propulsion was that my thighs would rotate and I couldn't carry anything on my lap. The research team added PA stimulation to the pattern. This pulled my knees together and made it easier to fill my lap with stuff for any distance wheeling.

The PA became the star for the lab visit in May. During the trunk stability testing in the FES Motion lab, we added the PA to the trunk functional stimulation pattern. Just the addition of these muscles added a volume of stability to the trunk pattern. Again, it brought my knees together and fulfilled a needed void to create a solid base for reaching. PA has now become a permanent staple to the menu of trunk stimulation patterns. But, the most noticeable impact was when we were tweaking the standing pattern.

During the May visit, we had many hours of tweaking the standing pattern and the technique for sit-to-stand. When I first arrived in the lab for stand training, the majority of my stands were less than perfect. In fact on the first day of training, I had more bad stands than good ones. This was a bit discouraging.

For a few standing attempts, I would twist my hips on the way up. On other tries, I would slide to the right. Yet on others, I would point my left toe and flex on my right heel. Between the twists, slides and foot movement, I looked like I was ready to join "Dancing with the Stars."

Tackling this issue, the research team had a tweaking option that might eliminate my dance routine, but would take at least two hours of programming. Essentially, they changed the stimulation sequence. In simple terms, during the ramp-up sequence for standing, they stimulated the hip extensor muscles prior to stimulating the quadriceps. After waiting for the new pattern, the first stand put a kibosh on the old sit-to-stand technique and my sit-to-stand become smoother.

But we were not done tweaking the standing pattern yet. An observation that I brought back to the lab was how I set up to stand with the crutches. Since I am a low level quadriplegic, I do not have any control of my trunk muscles. When I set up to stand with the crutches, I place my feet under my knees and scoot to the end of the wheelchair seat cushion. At the edge, I have a hard time sitting unsupported. To compensate for this, I have been turning on my back electrodes while sitting on the edge and setting up the crutches. Then I turn off the back stimulation and switch to the standing pattern. The therapist observed that with the back stimulation turned on, it is easier for me to get my shoulders over my knees for the sit-to-stand performance. Back to the programming board goes the engineer with my UECU.

The engineer did his magic. He gave me a new standing pattern. With one click of **Go**, my back electrodes engaged and with the second click the system went directly into the standing pattern.

This is all a new pattern for standing and, yes, we had to learn how to count all over again. I had to go back to Sesame Street and spend more time with Count von Count. But to our surprise, the PA came to my rescue. With this new pattern, the stimulation begins and as soon as the PA stimulation is on, my knees come together and it is time to make the transition

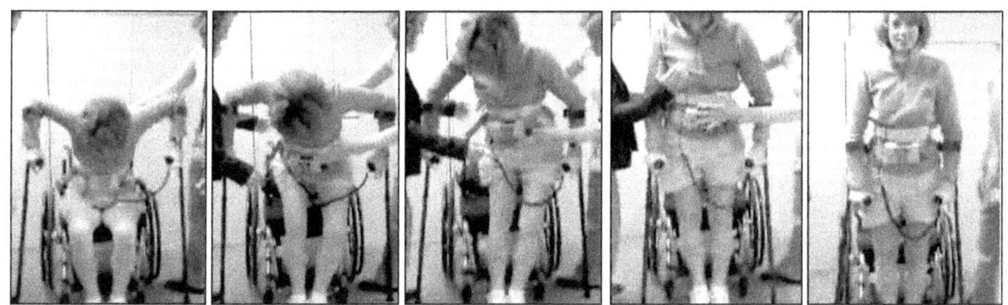

Standing from crutches.

from sit to stand. Like Dorothy from the Wizard of Oz clicking her heels together, I now click my knees together to stand up. I guess I need a new pair of red sneakers.

With this new standing pattern and the correct timing, getting up using crutches was almost effortless. I can now rely on the stimulation rather than brute arm strength. (I sure hope that doesn't negatively impact my arm-wrestling ability.) My sit to stand was still not perfect, but I was comfortable being independent and could now take more time to practice.

As I flew back to Florida reflecting on the May visit to the laboratory, I had a new appreciation for the post adductor muscles. It is an important muscle group that gets little respect.

Chapter 13: Going for Gold

Prove the technology in the real world. That is a duty of a research participant. With the world becoming a smaller place, traveling abroad is not outside the realm of this duty. As I return from Weymouth/Portland, United Kingdom after competing in the 2011 Sail for Gold Regatta, I reflect on the use of the new implanted system during my first travels outside North America.

During my previous visit to the lab, the technical team was challenged as to how the system may be recharged abroad. Apparently, there was quite a discussion, which revolved around the fact that the system recharges and operates at a specific voltage and it has never been tested abroad. In the end, I received a personal call from the technical lab manager (who also happens to be a sailor) advising me to use a voltage converter and to never use the system while the battery is recharging. As a compliant participant, I followed his orders.

In Weymouth/Portland, U.K. (on the southwest shore of England), our team rented a condo with a spectacular view of the racing area and the National Sailing Academy.

As we settled in for a week of racing, I needed to recharge the system after a long flight (more on that later). I was reminded of the Dry Bones children's song,

Oh dem plugs, dem plugs
the battery charger is connected to the plug adapter,
the plug adapter is connected to the voltage converter,
the voltage converter is connected to UK electrical adapter, and
the UK electrical adapter is connected to the wall unit,
Oh how scary it can be.

The moment of truth was at hand. I flicked the power switch on the battery charger to the **On** position. No lights, no power. My heart sank. Immediately, thoughts of how I could manage for 10 days without using the implanted system and taking stock of the remaining auxiliary battery power filled my head. *Okay, calm down and try to solve this problem.* I re-routed the electrical connections from the battery charger box to the wall unit. Next to the wall unit was a small breaker switch that was off. I flicked it to **On** and with a slight delay, power returned to the charger unit. I was back in business.

Aside from my daily standing routine, I put the system to the test using alternative functional patterns programmed by the research team. The two most used patterns were the **Glut Shift** pattern and the **Wheelchair Propulsion** pattern. The flight duration between Orlando, Florida and London is nearly eight hours. As a person with a mobility impairment, I sat in the airline seat for the full eight hours. With the exception of a few airplane types, there are no options to move around on long flights; not even to use the restroom. Sitting in the same position for that duration is a true pressure sore risk. During this long flight, I used the **Glut Shift** pattern to provide much needed relief. This pattern stimulates the gluteus maximus, hamstrings, and the post adductors, alternating between the right and left sides. The stimulation helps to increase blood flow and muscle contraction to the critical areas that are vulnerable to pressure sores. After using it for this long flight, the batteries, including the auxiliary batteries were nearly dead.

The other pattern that I used frequently during this trip was the **Wheelchair Propulsion** pattern. In the lab, we discovered that this pattern does not increase propulsion speed but dramatically decreases the effort that I exert to propel my wheelchair. The pattern stimulates the gluteus maximus, gluteus medius, post adductors, hamstrings, erector spinae, and quadratus. The combination makes my body more solid in the wheelchair seat.

As I mentioned, our team rented a condo while in Weymouth/ Portland. The condo was approximately one mile from the sailing venue and it was on a small hill along the waterfront. The daily trek to the sailing center had a few inclines and descends along the waterfront footpath. On my first day, I attempted the trek with no stimulation. I learned my lesson and did not do that again. Every morning, I would listen to the song of the day, turn the **Wheelchair Propulsion** pattern on, and proceed along my path to the sailing center. After sailing each day, I would reverse the process. I could make it all the way back to the condo parking lot, but there was one hill where I needed assistance. The final incline was so high that regardless of the stimulation, it was very difficult to propel up the hill.

On this trip abroad, the test patterns were pushed to their limits in the real world. To me, they have proven their value as a user of the implanted system. The system provided much-needed pressure relief during a very long flight and it provided the needed stability to propel my wheelchair on my one-mile daily trek. I'm sure other users will have different experiences, but for me the patterns proved themselves in the real world.

Paying the Consequences

After returning from the U.K., I was pretty excited about my real-world experiences with the new patterns programmed into the system. The **Wheelchair Propulsion** pattern made it easier to wheel between the condo and the sailing venue. The **Glut Shift** pattern helped reduce the pressure while sitting in an airline seat for nearly eight hours. And the **Trunk Control** pattern aided my daily functions in a condo that was not quite wheelchair-accessible.

That is all great. But each of those patterns excludes one important muscle group, the quadriceps. I failed to recognize it earlier and after returning home, I paid the consequences. Unfortunately, this issue did not surface until I was back home and returned to standing with the crutches.

You see, during competition and even the few days leading into it, there is not much time for activities away from sailing. We typically spent five hours on the water with at least one hour on either end for boat work. Add on weather briefings, coach's reviews, an occasional protest, dinner, and a shower and I'm done for the day. The exception is a weather delay; and we all know how reliable the weather is! In fact, I've been caught falling asleep while exercising with the system after being on the water all day. Unfortunately, there is not much time for anything else.

Standing is one of the few patterns that stimulate the quadriceps. This is a critical muscle group for standing. The quads are the powerhouse I depend on to move from the seated to the standing position. Alas, they are also the first to fatigue and demand a rest. I get lazy standing with the walker, since I can rely more on my own arm strength to get me up. On this last trip to the U.K., Tim was not with me so I brought the walker for standing. Yes, I was lazy and had little standing time.

When I returned home to begin standing with crutches again, my quads just weren't up for the task. Back to the gym—actually, back to weight-lifting. With the need to strengthen the quad muscles, I started a daily routine of leg lifts with ankle weights. Beginning with five pounds, I gradually built up to 10 pounds with three sets of 10 lifts. About a week later, I once again had the strength to stand with the crutches. It is amazing how quickly the muscles weaken when they are not used.

As I prepared to return to the U.K. for a second round of sailing competition (a.k.a. regatta) at the 2011 Disabled Sailing World Championship, I was more aware of the consequences if I slacked off with standing. Plus, this time I'd have Tim with me and he definitely will not let me get lazy.

Applying the Test Patterns

After returning from my two-month trip to the United Kingdom for competition, I paid a much-needed visit to the FES lab in Cleveland. This was an opportunity to use the new implanted system, along with various functional patterns, to see how they can benefit life for a person living with a spinal cord injury. Aside from standing, while traveling abroad I found the trunk control, wheelchair propulsion, and pressure sore prevention patterns to be incredibly useful.

Now it's time to get back in the lab and round out the various research studies included in the overall clinical trial that I

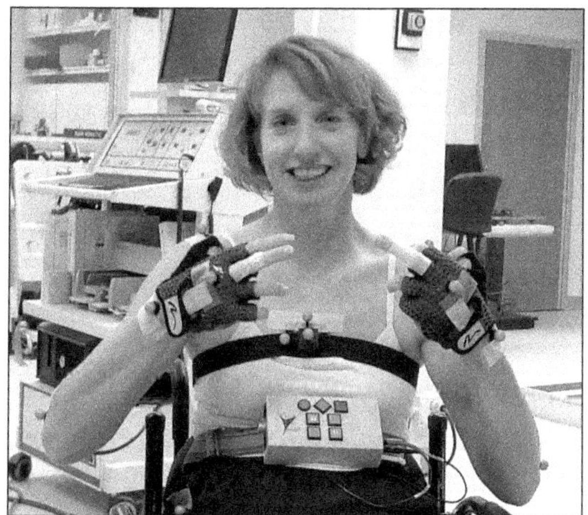
In the Motion Study Lab

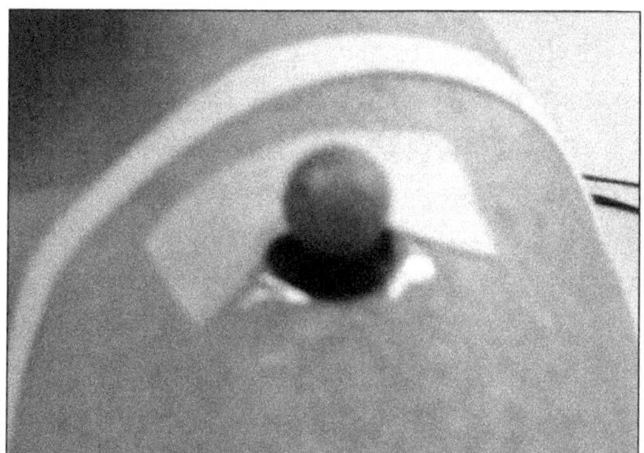
Reflector balls placed on my body

joined almost a year ago. The August 2011 visit consisted of five days in the lab, broken by a weekend in Cleveland. The activities over the course of the five-day visit fell into three categories: cuff electrode experiments, trunk control testing, and stand and transfer training.

Job one is the cuff electrode experiments. As we've seen, the cuff electrode is a small spiral consisting of four channel contacts. Each channel contact may be programmed independently. This device is surgically implanted and surrounds the fermoral nerve to control the muscles in the quadriceps.

This type of electrode has been implanted into only a few participants in the standing program. The research team is trying to understand how this electrode design improves use of the system to control the complex group of muscles comprising the thigh. The electrode targets three of the four main muscles in the quad group controlled by the femoral nerve: the vastus lateralis, vastus intermedius, and the vastus medialis.

One research project studies how oscillating patterns between the four channels in each cuff electrode can delay fatigue and provide longer standing durations. The current standing pattern stimulates the quadricep muscles to a full contraction with no resting times while standing. As the powerhouse of the human leg, this muscle group plays a critical role in going from sit to stand. It is also typically the first muscle to fatigue; requiring the user to sit and rest the muscle. In theory, by introducing an oscillation pattern to the stimulation, the system will allow rest time for muscles, thus providing longer standing durations. So how does this apply to the standing system?

Over the course of the year, I spent countless hours on the dynamometer to gather data and guide the engineers who are designing the oscillation patterns. After some final testing, it was time to try the patterns in actual standing. I first tried to stand using the oscillation patterns with no data-gathering equipment but simply a walker and the research therapist. I would go from sit to stand using my typical standing pattern. After I settled into a solid stance, we tested each of the oscillation patterns. After observing how the patterns impacted the quads we stopped to allow me to sit and discuss the experience. With this information in hand, it was back for more dynamometer work.

Now, it was time to gather data while using the standing system that included the new oscillation patterns. In the lab, there are a set of parallel bars and force plates on the floor. Both are wired to collect data while standing to evaluate the weight distribution between my arms and my legs. The test method consists of standing using the oscillation pattern for one minute or until my legs fatigue, whichever is longer. With the therapist guarding my knees and the engineer holding the external control unit with the experimental patterns, I stood inside the parallel bars. Each stand was only for about a minute, but long enough to gather the data the research team needed.

Back to the drawing board to understand how the cuff electrodes used in the standing system can be optimized for my particular nerves and muscles. The research team needed more time and information to continue to explore this new concept. It's an incremental learning process that requires patience and the ability to deal with unexpected results. That's the nature of research. It's important to remember that we learn something new that moves us forward with every experiment, regardless of the outcome.

Staying in My Seat

Standing is a grand gesture; it offers me the ability to escape the wheelchair. However, there are other features of the implanted system that can also provide valuable functions that may not be as glamorous and are often overlooked when discussing the system. As a person with a high-level spinal cord injury, I lack voluntary control of the core or trunk muscles. Gaining function of these muscles will not only help with seated posture but use of the upper body to improve daily activities while I'm in the wheelchair.

As a recipient of the implanted neural prosthesis, I have also been eligible to participate in a research program to improve seated posture and trunk control. The research team was investigating the value of using selected electrodes that control my hip and spine muscles for trunk stability. Over several months, the team had been conducting a variety of experiments to collect data on how stimulating these muscles can help improve the function of someone while they're sitting.

The first functional experiment was reaching ability with and without stimulation of the trunk. Here, we used the Motion Study Laboratory at the Louis Stokes VA Hospital. This lab uses motion-sensing cameras to build images of movement. With a therapy mat on center stage within a sea of cameras, the research team draped a long string of reflective beads from the ceiling, representing typical low shelf and table heights above the floor. The team then strategically placed reflector balls onto my body; elbows, shoulders, sternum, and a small pole on the lumbar spine.

With the stage set, I sat on the edge of the mat and performed randomly selected tasks of reaching forward with and without stimulation and with empty or weighted boxes. For each task, a student intern would list the required task, ie. "Low target, with stimulation, weighted box," and the therapist would hand me the proper box while monitoring my movements. This went on for an hour. Yes, I got bored after the first 15 minutes. To liven it up, the therapist and I would guess what the next task sequence would be. Nine times out of 10, I would guess wrong.

The other function to test was wheelchair propulsion. As a low-level quadriplegic (C6-7), using a manual wheelchair has its challenges. However, there are many health benefits to choosing a manual wheelchair over a power wheelchair for someone with my level of function. But what if stimulation can provide a means to propel my wheelchair with less effort and less energy?

Our experiments started off by replacing my current wheelchair wheels with a data collection set. The first of four experiments was in the Motion Study Lab at the VA. To capture my motion while I propelled my wheelchair, reflective balls were placed all over my body. When it was all set up, I looked pretty funny.

During this experiment, I would wheel across the "stage" at a constant pace, with and without the trunk stimulation. As you can image, wheeling back and forth, back and forth, gets a little monotonous. To keep us entertained, I would play around with the images on the screens between experiments; I found I could make swimming motions or dance moves. In the end, stimulation dramatically changed my posture in the wheelchair. With stimulation, I have a very straight and proper posture. Without stimulation, my posture is slouched or "slinky down." We returned the reflector balls and headed out into the real world for more experiments.

The 100-meter dash was next. The research team found a straight and level stretch in the hospital. The test was to propel my wheelchair as fast as I could for 100 meters with and without stimulation. The student intern was further up the 100 meter course from me to keep the path clear and my mom was staged further up the course to do the same.

Over the course of the experiments, there were groups of nurses and therapists that became near misses as I flew past them. But the best was during one experiment, when a staff member unknowingly parked a lunch cart in the middle of the hallway and put the brake on. As I got closer and closer to the cart, it was almost inevitable that I would hit it. My mom attempted to move it but couldn't get the brake disengaged. Calling for help, she summoned the student intern who used all of his strength to push the cart aside...it was a close call and I narrowly avoided sending Jell-O and soup flying all over the hallway.

Speed tests done.

The final wheelchair propulsion tests were ramps. Urgh! One ramp was carpeted and had a lower slope and the other was cement with a higher slope. For both ramp tests, I propelled up the ramp with and without stimulation. The cement ramp is in the walkway to the new wing of the VA hospital. In this wing, there is minimal people traffic and the experiments were completed with little fanfare. On the other hand, the carpeted ramp is in the walkway from the parking garage to the main atrium of the hospital. Now, those experiments were much more...entertaining.

As any manual wheelchair user knows, navigating a ramp

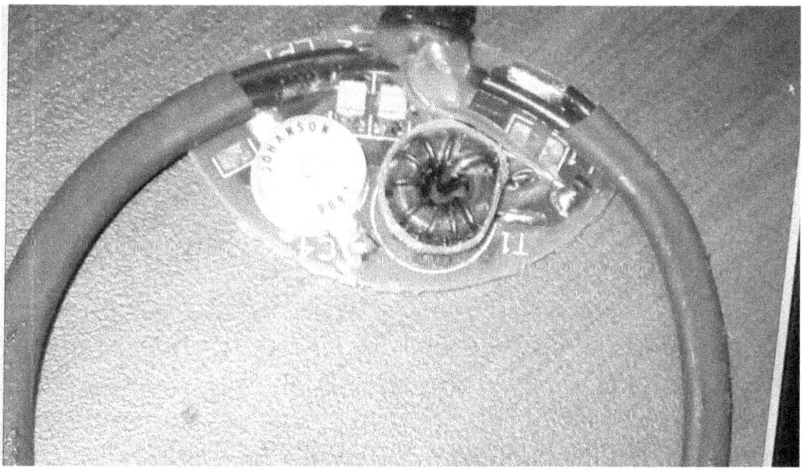

Circuitry of external coil, which communicates with the implanted receiver

with carpeting is not an easy task. My mom and the intern did a great job of keeping people to one side on the ramp. The expressions on the faces of people passing by were mixed; some perplexed, others inquisitive—some even cheered me on. During one of our resting times, the therapist commented about how she could beat my time. Not to pass up a dare, I popped out of my wheelchair and handed my wheelchair over to her. "Here, go ahead. You try it."

Armed with my wheelchair and the challenge on the table, the therapist took my wheelchair to the bottom of the ramp. She beat my time by almost half. "What! No, way. There must be error." Second time around, she did it again. What a Wonder Woman! But it wasn't over yet. The student intern, who happened to be on the Case Western Reserve University swim team, decided he wanted in on this impromptu wheelchair competition. His proposal: He can beat both times using a hospital transport wheelchair; those heavy, inefficient depot wheelchairs. Convinced there was no way he can beat our times, the therapist and I took him up on the challenge. Pushing as fast as he could, the intern beat even my therapist's time. Ouch!

After being smoked by the therapist and the 20 year-old student intern, I was crushed. Of course, I wanted to blame the technology. In the end, it was all for good fun. But the reality is that the evidence is mounting that trunk stimulation may make life as a quadriplegic in a manual wheelchair much more functional. The other reality is that I need to get back to the gym!

Troubleshooting

Trust. It's a fragile emotion. It's hard to earn and easy to lose. The physical therapist hadn't released me for independent standing with crutches because of trust—I needed to earn it. The therapist needed to trust that I would be successful and safe while standing with crutches and I had not demonstrated that yet. But trust goes both ways. I needed to trust that when I tape the coils to my skin and activate the standing system, it will work. Most recently, my trust of the implanted system was tested.

With this system, there are implanted components and external components, each of which need to communicate with each other. That communication is called coupling. The external coil must communicate with the internally implanted receiver. If that coupling relationship is compromised, the system does not operate properly.

The coupling problem persisted. Time to troubleshoot. I tried re-taping the coils, using different coils, adding auxiliary batteries—all the tools at my disposal—but with no success. Then, the "what-ifs" started to surface. What if the UECU is bad and they don't have a backup from the technical lab? What if I need more power from the system but we're already near maximum capacity? What if the implanted receiver has gone bad? At one point, Tim and I no longer trusted the system for standing. But to feed my addiction to standing, Tim would spot me while I stood with a walker, a task that was once a piece of cake for me. We were losing trust in the system and I was quickly losing my independence. Time to call in the mechanics.

During my August 2011 visit to Cleveland, coupling was the first thing to troubleshoot. Consulting with the program engineer, I handed him all four coils and the UECU, explaining the situation. After some testing, he came back with the results. The UECU tested fine but only two of the four coils were functioning on the test system.

The coils are a small component that takes a daily beating due to having tape applied and removed and due to constantly being subjected to mechanical stresses with movement of my body. Sometimes they can malfunction due to daily use. The research program recognized these shortcomings and worked on several ideas to improve the reliability of the coils.

The quick solution was to issue new coils to me. Safety is a high priority so the team added a coupling testing pattern. Here I can connect the coil to the UECU, press a button, and the system will beep if there is not a proper coupling. The engineers added an additional safety feature. If the quality of the coupling declined, it would first deactivate only some electrodes rather than all of them. Now, before taping the coils to my skin, I could test the system to reassure that I have proper coil placement before taping them down for the day. I called it my trust-building button. The issue was elevated to the technical lab for the engineers to research additional solutions.

Dance Moves

But our troubleshooting was still upon us. Over the 12 years of using the standing system, I had been the participant with the clumsy dance moves. When I first started standing with the eight-channel system, I would get a spasm in my hips. My hips would shake from side to side like I was playing with a hula hoop. Like clockwork, my first few minutes of standing would induce a hips spasm and I would hula. We even added a fictitious "Hula" button to my UECU. Over time, the spasm went away and I lost my hula move.

More recently, I had been having some difficultly getting from sit to stand using the crutches. During this most recent visit, I asked the research team to observe what was happening to help troubleshoot the issue. What they observed: As I stand up, my left toe points upward and my right foot flexes and kicks out. The engineer mimicked the move and labeled it the "Irish jig." Yet another dance move!

Unfortunately, this dance move was not functional so the physical therapist began to work her troubleshooting methods to help find the culprit. I transferred onto the therapy mat and we began checking each individual muscle group. The gluteus medius is the muscle in the hip that scissors the leg out. When we tested the left gluteus medius, it almost tossed the therapist off her square stool. I guess there is a little power in that electrode. Also during this check, we discovered that the post adductor (the muscle that pulls the legs together) contraction was not strong enough to offset the contraction from the gluteus medius. Suspecting that this offset was the culprit, we turned the post adductor up to get a stronger contraction.

The culprit for the left foot planterflexion (pointing up) was the hamstring. By turning it down, we found that we could decrease the contraction to stop the spillover to the foot. It still amazes me how the intricacies of muscles work together in the human body.

With her tweaking over, the therapist gave her recommendation to the program engineer. He went back to his office for some system programming and returned with a new program loaded into the UECU. Using the walker, I tried a stand to see how the latest adjustments integrated together in the standing pattern. I pressed the button, activated the system, and stood up out of the chair. The left toe pointing was gone and the right foot flexion was no more. With that, I lost my Irish Jig dance move.

But we discovered another consequence of our actions. While we turned up the stimulation to the post adductors, my legs were stuck together as if by a magnet. The contraction was so strong that the therapist couldn't separate my feet. To go from sit to stand, the strong contraction was good but for standing and transferring the result was not favorable. The engineers tweaked the system to get the best of both.

Sit to stand was now a dream, nearly effortless. Standing with crutches was much easier and now just a matter of practicing the technique and re-building my trust of the system.

Despite all my nitpicking of the system, we shouldn't lose sight of what has been accomplished. A person with paralysis who had been committed to life in a wheelchair can now stand up under her own muscle power. That is a pretty incredible accomplishment. It's bigger than my body.

A Spring in My Step

The protocol of the research program is for me to stand and transfer using a walker. With the old system, I could stand with a walker but it required a lot of arm strength and I could only stand for a short period of time. Prior to receiving the upgrade, I was standing with only five of the original eight-electrode system. One electrode was not operating and two others provided a low-level muscle contraction that was not functional. After receiving the upgrade, I was back up standing and transferring with a walker. That was a piece of cake.

Beyond the expectations of the original system design, I have been standing with crutches. During the August 2011 visit to the Cleveland laboratory, we started to experiment with transfers using crutches and the standing system. The first attempts were difficult. Once again, crutches have proven to be a more fickle ambulation tool.

The particular set of crutches I was using was not very dependable. The physical therapist was the first to observe the equipment issue. You see, the crutches that I used were Loftstrand crutches, which feature a spring at the base. In theory this can help with propulsion and perhaps going from sit to stand. In reality, the springs were the obstacle and the source of instability. With just a few centimeters difference, I could not get the clearance off the crutches to lift my feet off the ground.

Ever resourceful, members of the team contacted the supplier of the crutches and ordered a new base without the springs. Timing was not on our side, as this discovery occurred during the last day of my lab time. The new bases would have to be shipped to my home in Florida.

Within a week, they arrived. Not one to waste time, I opened them up and switched out the bases. With Tim's supervision, I tried to stand with the new equipment. The first few attempts to stand were not pretty. In fact some attempts had to be aborted.

After a while, though, taking the spring out of my step made a big difference. Over the next several days, the results of my sit to stand attempts yielded more successful independent stands than aborted attempts. I was on the verge of finally getting the hang of this. But the true test will be to prove it to the physical therapist during my next visit to the lab.

Getting Ready for Release

The test protocols were coming to a close and I would soon be released from the program. What does getting released mean?

Getting released from a clinical trial involving an implanted device is a bit unique. For a pharmaceutical trial, you just stop taking the drug, respond to a few surveys, and then go on your merry way. (I've been involved in a few drug trials). With a medical device, it's not that easy. In fact, it is much more complex.

The option of taking the experimental device out, like discontinuing a medication, is ludicrous. The option to stop using the device is hard to accept.

But some in the industry and regulatory agencies advocate administering an implanted medical device trial like a drug trial. How can we in good conscience restore function to people with paralysis and then take it away in the name of science? After gaining function back at the press of a button and integrating it into your life, taking the option away again is like being spinal cord injured all over again. Sometimes I question if regulators, funding agencies, grant reviewers, and other folks in the medical device industry understand that simple fact.

With this in mind, there is a reason I have stayed with the Principal Investigator and his team working at the Cleveland FES Center. They understand the dependence on restored function that their participants acquire. They are truly dedicated to the participants in their programs. Once I am released from the program, the frequent travel between Florida and Ohio will cease. However, the team will conduct a six-month and a one-year follow up. They will continue to collect data from the UECU. Every three months, there will be a transport case on my doormat for the data swap. If I encounter any problems, the team will continue to be available as long as the Principal Investigator is able to secure and maintain research funding for this and other projects.

Most importantly, I can continue to use the system in my daily life. But in research, as in life, there are no guarantees. At some point in the future, the funding for this research project may evaporate. Then what? If our current medical system in the U.S. remains the same, there is no long-term interest for anyone to receive implanted medical devices from research projects. But how can commercial devices be developed if there are no pioneers willing to be research participants?

Sure, it is a risk and a personal responsibility that I willingly and knowingly undertook. It was communicated to me in no uncertain terms in the many legal documents associated with the research project. However, an implanted device is not like testing a beta version of the latest tablet PC, where you can send it back or toss it out without any real loss except some time and maybe a few dollars.

At some point, the research community and the agencies who fund investigational implanted medical devices need to address the issue of long-term users of early stage technologies. Look at how much we have learned in just 12 months of using this device in this research program. Now, imagine what we can learn in five years or 10. As I prepare to be released, this issue resonates in my mind. In the meantime, I'll enjoy the use of the system and remain reassured by the dedication and support of the Principal Investigator and his team at the FES Center.

On my final visit to the Cleveland FES Center, I was in for some final testing. The investigators took the opportunity to try some proof of concept experiments with the pressure relief and trunk control patterns. The most important part of the visit was standing with the crutches. This was the final goal to reach before signing the release papers for the trial.

With that in mind, Tim and I worked hard before my final visit to Cleveland. The physical therapist is notoriously difficult to impress but we also understand that she always has safety as a first priority. Over the course of this visit, my only focus was to do an independent stand with the crutches. In the lab with the therapist advising, I did three "good" independent stands. With

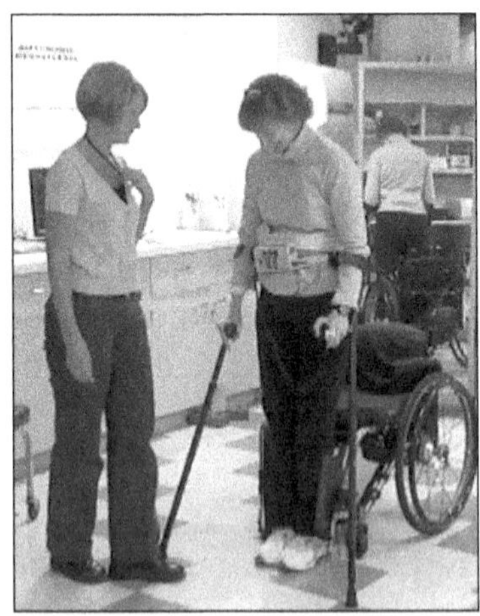

My "impressive" stand

those behind me, we set up a mirror and a camera to get the full view of an independent stand. The next attempt, I would stand with no assistance. With the press of **Go** and the cameras rolling, my stand was unsuccessful. I tried a few more times, but they were unsuccessful. It must be fatigue, I thought, so we took a short break to let the muscles recover.

We reconvened in the lab. I told the therapist that this is it so stand back. I pressed **Go** and got a perfect stand with the crutches. We even caught on video the therapist saying "She is very stable. Very impressive." That was all I needed; mission accomplished.

Chapter 14: End of a Journey

Reflecting on the progress over the previous 14 months, I'm amazed at how far we have come. In August 2010, a medical device was implanted into my body. Over the following year, the system was tested, tweaked, and reprogrammed. Along the way, I gained a free back massage, an easier way to propel my wheelchair, and the ability to stand and transfer for functional uses.

There have been countless hours in the lab and numerous email exchanges. In this book, I've mentioned the surgeons, the engineers, and the therapists. But in reality there is an army of people working on developing this device. They are the ones that we don't see, like programmers in the technical lab, developers tweaking the equipment, students testing the experimental design, nurses giving exceptional care, and administrators managing the array of paperwork. They have ownership in this system just as much as those on the front lines who work with the participants.

There are also the hidden heroes. I've been fortunate to have an incredible support network. My husband, Tim, has sacrificed so much to help me from surgery recovery to functional use. He has become harder on me than the therapist, but I love it. My in-laws, are loyal cat-sitters and have helped with the cleaning while I'm away. My sister and her family have hosted me in their home for the many visits to Cleveland with countless meals and scheduling arrangements. This book wouldn't be complete without recognizing my mom. What a trooper; meeting me at the airport in the wee-hours of the morning, driving me between hospitals and laboratories, waiting while I have meetings and tests, and pitching in when the research team needs a hand. And the cookies! The research team will forever be spoiled by my mom's cookies. Over the course of time, she has become a member of the research team. She is a true hidden hero.

Of course, money makes the world work. The research project would not be possible without the funding agencies who believed in the concept and supported this research team: Case Western Reserve University, MetroHealth Medical Center, National Institutes of Neurological Disorders and Stroke, and the Veterans Administration Research and Development. Yes, this project is partially funded by the VA. Although I am not a veteran, being a participant is one way that I can give back to our wounded warriors living with spinal cord injuries. It is my hope that one day, they will benefit from the discoveries of this research.

As I reflect on this experience, it is so easy to get used to the technology and integrate it into my daily routine. After a while there is never a second thought about turning on the system for a pressure relief, pressing a button to get trunk control, or having the option to stand and transfer. When I take the coils off and put the UECU on the charger, I'm reminded of the way I was left after the spinal cord injury, minus all these new bionic functions. It is a reminder to appreciate the technology.

This experience was not just a discovery of the technology but also a discovery of myself. I learned to appreciate the power of music and images catering to the importance of mental preparation. Quoting lyrics to songs often helps me define an experience and describe it more eloquently. The images that were taped to the walls of my hospital room and helped me overcome the post-surgical pain are now staples of the Clinical Research Unit.

I've learned patience for others and for myself. The time waiting to properly set up an experiment or the time to allow the body to heal properly demonstrated the power of patience. The hours spent during experiments repeated in order to achieve reliability forced me to find ways to keep the team (and myself) entertained.

I've learned that the process of experimentation is never straightforward. I appreciate the importance of flexibility in design—and redesign—in order to get the best outcome. I recognize that discovery comes with successful trials but also from failure. Each is a critical part of research—and any growing experience for that matter.

Even after the Wow factor from the initial stand has worn thin, I find that I've grown more demanding of the system. I expect it to work every time the system is booted up. And, it does. Daily use transforms from a nice option to a necessity in life as a quadriplegic living independently.

Music has become intertwined in this experience. Every time I draft a journal entry, themed music is in the periphery. As I write this final chapter, these lyrics from John Mayer resonate in my ears:

This is a call to the color blind. This is an I.O.U...

cause I'm bigger than my body gives me credit for...

What a great way to sum up this experience. The research is about more than my ability to stand using my own muscles. It is functional recovery after a spinal cord injury, even for people like me who are more than 10 years post-injury.

Finally, this book can't be closed without thanking all the readers and followers of my journey. The messages of encouragement, gracious cheers, and heartfelt notes have helped me along the way. I am still amazed at even the silent readers.

I hope this effort has helped build an understanding of the human experience and the required commitments of clinical trials. I am not the only one to have participated in the exciting world of scientific advancement, nor will I be the last. Mine is but one small contribution I can make to the evolution of technology and the continuing effort to improve life for people living with spinal cord injury.

Thank you for the experience.

Epilogue: My Journey to London 2012

While I was in an acute rehabilitation hospital in Concord, NH, Jill Gravink from Northeast Passage paid us a visit. She came with an elaborate video along with equipment of adaptive sports, including a mountain bike and a road handcycle. While showing us the video, she spoke of the various adaptive sports such as snow skiing, waterskiing, and more. She is a certified recreational therapist and emphasized the importance of sport in the rehabilitation process. Apparently, my physical therapist explained to her that I was involved with outdoor activities prior to my accident and thought that recreation would be helpful to me.

After her presentation, I looked at her in frustration.

"Thank you, but I'm still learning how to get dressed and pee. Recreation is the last thing on my priority list."

My intent was not to be rude, but I could not understand why she came and how recreation can possibly help with the devastation of a spinal cord injury.

Weekend in Tewksbury

Months later after my transition home, we received a brochure about a waterski weekend in Tewksbury, MA. Tim and I discussed attending and I brought the idea to my neurologist. At the time, I was still wearing a brace to stabilize my neck, which contained surgically placed titanium wire. With hesitancy, my neurologist approved of our attendance but stressed that I may not participate in waterskiing. By doing that, I would put my neck at risk and potentially induce more damage. We decided to go for one day. We were not ready to take on the unknown task of staying overnight in a hotel.

We arrived at the park in late morning. This was the first time we were exposed to a group of people in wheelchairs outside the hospital setting. They were waterskiing, doing floor-to-chair transfers, performing wheelies, swimming in the lake and going out boating. In that day, I learned more than in the past several months of rehabilitation. Just being able to watch how others tackled the daily challenges that kept me from "normal" life was enlightening. Now, we understand the impact of recreational therapy.

Fast-forward a year; we received another postcard for an outdoor event. This time it was organized by Vermont Ski and Sport for a water sporting event on Mallets Bay in Colchester, VT. The event would include kayaking, sailing, and swimming. We decided to try it and spend the weekend in our beloved Vermont while visiting some old friends. This was the first time I was back in a sailboat since my injury. Ironically, the first boat I sailed was a Sonar. Years later, it would be my preferred boat to race. This Sonar was situated with a seat near the stern with a ring that lowered around me. That ring was attached to the rudder for steering. The system was designed by Gene Hinkel of St. Petersburg, FL; he was the father of Paralympic Sailing. We enjoyed the weekend of reuniting with sailboats.

Prior to my spinal cord injury, Tim's family would cruise on the family sailboat, the Destiny. She is a 1969 35-foot Allied Seabreeze. Encouraged by the report from our weekend on Mallets Bay, Tim's dad designed a way to transfer me into the sailboat. It was innovated by the talents of Tim's parents. Joe created a series of lines that attached to the main halyard while Betty sewed an over-sized pair of Wrangler Jean cut off to shorts and with connection grommets. When pulled together, the system would use the designs of the boat to gently lift me from my wheelchair and onto the boat. With this tool, we were again able to cruise New England and return to the vacation times we enjoyed in the past while creating new ones.

The World of Racing

Three years after my injury and after being released from the Cleveland FES Center program for the initial eight-channel implanted system, Tim and I moved to Tampa Bay, FL. A family friend, Pat Seidenspinner, introduced us to the St. Petersburg Sailing Center. This facility had been renovated to be completely wheelchair accessible in preparation for hosting the 2001 International Federation of Disabled Sailing World Championship. It would become our new playground.

In 2001, I was new to the sport of sailboat racing and paid a visit during the World Championship. Once again, there were several people in wheelchairs with spinal cord injuries, limb amputations, degenerative diseases, and other disorders. It was my first introduction to sailboat racing and the adaptations that come along with the sport. More important, it was my first introduction to a sport where I could compete with or against my able-bodied friends.

Over the next several weeks, I would be introduced to the 2.4mR boat, the single-handed Paralympic keelboat. My first regatta was the Disabled/Open Regatta in the spring of 2002. At the time, Tom Brown was participating in the same regatta and the same 2.4mR class. He would later win the silver medal at the 2004 Paralympic Games. At this particular regatta, he would lap me on the race course; sometimes twice. I was so slow and new to the sport. I was soaked with saltwater, bruised and full of smiles, but I didn't care that I was in last place. It was fun and refreshing to know that I could sail a boat on my own.

For the next 10 years, Tim and I would take on the task of learning to race sailboats and find ways to adapt the sailboat to my specific disability. We would later meet Gene Hinkel, the man who designed the seat installed in the Sonar that I sailed in Vermont. Gene and Joe, along with Derek at JTR Marine, worked with us to create adaptive equipment to allow me to be competitive against fully able-bodied teams in the 23-foot Sonar. In the end, sailboat racing was a sport that Tim and I could compete together or against each other. We met amazing people along the way: Ed Sherman, Colin Park, John Jennings, Charley Morgan, Betsy Alison, and so many others.

A new boat was introduced to the Paralympic Sailing scene, the 18-foot SKUD. It debuted at the 2008 Paralympics in Beijing. The SKUD-18 would be the first Paralympic boat to fly a spinnaker, the big colorful balloon sail. After some prodding by sailing coaches, I teamed up with long time friend and bronze medalist from the 2004 Paralympic Games, Jean-Paul (JP) Creignou. At the time, we did not own a boat; however, Magnus Lilejedahl of Team Paradise loaned us a boat to use for competition. After just two months of training, JP and I competed in the 2010 Miami Olympic Classes Regatta. We finished in second place. That was the launch of a two -year campaign to reach the 2012 Paralympic Games in London.

During those two years, we would gather a large team of talent to help us. Our team would spend endless hours on the docks, on the water, and in the boat park. The hours logged turned into blood, sweat, and tears of commitment for a dream to represent Team USA at the 2012 Paralympic Games in London. We would need to pull together an elaborate plan of training, travel, and competition. Tim and I put aside commitments in our lives and focused on this one goal.

Qualifying Regattas

Our first challenge was to win the U.S. Paralympic trials process, which included a series of regattas against other U.S. teams. This was not a simple challenge and was accompanied by unforeseen drama along the way. One of our key strategic decisions was to hire Ian Clingan, as our personal sailing coach. He had been the coach for Great Britain's SKUD-18 team and was available for hire. He was our guide to development outside of the scope of the U.S. Sailing structure.

The trials process consisted of two regattas. Whichever team had the best collective score at the two events would win the honor to represent Team USA at the 2012 Paralympic Games. The first event would be the World Championship in Port Charlotte, FL. The venue was just 90 minutes south of our home base in St. Petersburg. The venue was on a river and learning the waters was imperative. For a major competitive event such as this, we prepared our equipment, learned the race course, and perfected the techniques. We worked on our bodies and minds to prepare for competition, but sometimes you can't prepare for everything.

The day before competition, I received a call from our veterinarian. Our beloved Maine-coon cat, Baxter, had just passed away. For the prior two months, we did everything we could to save him; three blood transfusions, CAT scans, x-rays, and biological tests that turned into hours at the vet. In the end, we couldn't save him. I received the call four hours before I was to report to the docks for the practice race. I never thought that I would be so attached to a pet.

In the back of our minds, Tim and I knew it was coming, but we did not want to accept it. At the time, I could not even mention it without tears flowing. I cried my eyes dry in the bathroom of our rented apartment, composed myself and left for the docks. At that point, the importance of mental preparation became clear. Later at the Paralympic Games, my fellow Australian competitor lost her mother during the event. Every day, she arrived at the docks ready to compete. If I were in her shoes, I would be an emotional wretch. I will always admire her for her mental discipline while facing a deeply emotional event. As for the regatta, we went on to finish in second place at the regatta; our closest U.S. competition was four places back. One more event to go.

With a week break, the team reconvened in Miami for the 2012 Olympic Classes Regatta (MOCR). It would be the second event of the trials process to win a ticket to the 2012 Paralympic Games. Miami is the backyard to our key U.S. competitors and we needed to just stay ahead and compete fairly to seal the deal. With a variety of conditions from warm, sunny, and light winds to rain, cool, and heavy winds, our team finished the regatta in third place. But final placement in the regatta didn't matter at this point. What mattered was that we won the ticket. We won the U.S. trials process and would be part of the U.S. 2012 Paralympic Sailing Team.

It was a big seat to fill. For the 2008 Paralympic Games in Beijing, the U.S., led by Nick Scandone with crew Maureen McKinnon-Tucker, won the Gold medal in the SKUD-18 class. Nick was a legendary sailor who died of ALS just four months after receiving the Gold medal.

It was February 2012 and we had six months to prepare for the Games. Life went on hold. The only focus was preparation for the Games. Every day there were hours dedicated to the mission. Family members stepped in to give a helping hand. Friends gave us support and guidance. Our final mission: make it to the podium at the 2012 Paralympics Games in London. The six months went by in a flash.

In August, 2012, we arrived at the competition venue, the National Sailing Academy in Weymouth/Portland UK, with the support of our family, friends, and country. At that point, training was over; it was time to perform and have fun doing it. The competition would be a series of 11 races. The top three performers would be honored with podium positions.

In the first race of a long series, JP and I had a good start

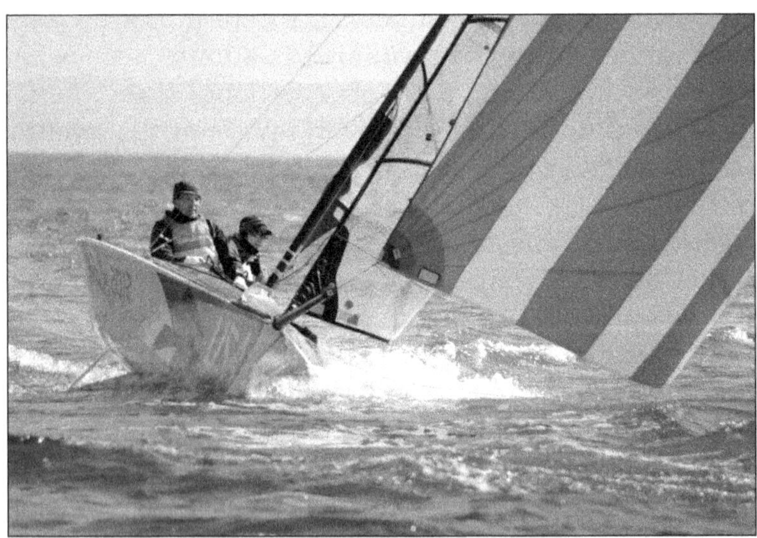

Downwind in Weymouth/Portland (Photo courtesy of International Federation of Disabled Sailing)

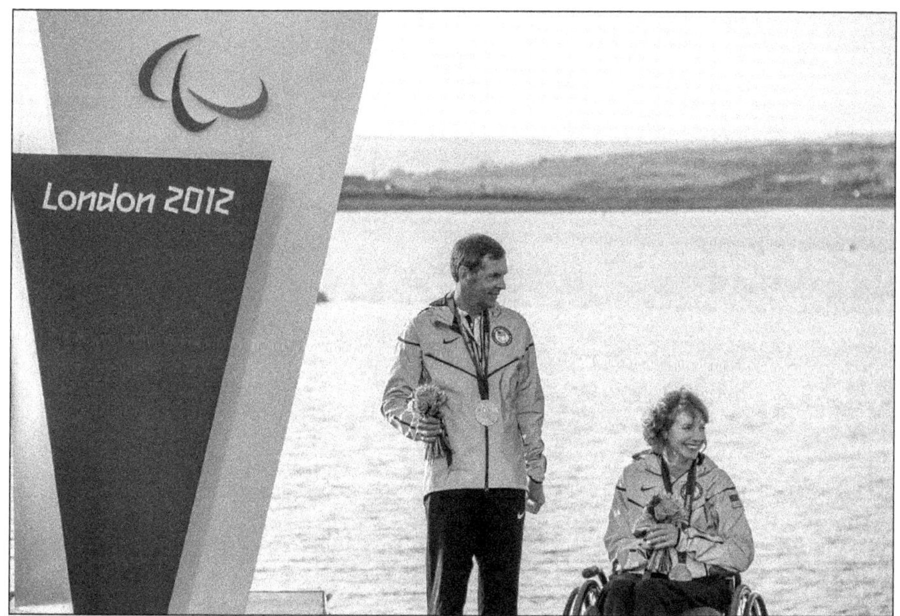

JP and I accept our silver medals. (Photo courtesy of U.S. Sailing)

off the line, but things unraveled for us. Shortly after launch a line got wrapped around our steering system; we basically had no steering. After four very slow tacks, we finally released the line and had our steering back. We rounded the first mark in dead last place, but we fought back to finish the race in third place. The next series of races were nail biters with close competition. Friends and family were watching with binoculars on the hill and over the Internet on the GPS tracking system. We fought our way among fierce competition. On the last day of the event, we finished in second place. We made the podium bringing home a silver medal for Team USA.

Looking back, it was not just JP and I in the boat. It was our family members, dedicated friends, and cheering supporters. Even though there were only two people on the boat, we had many more people racing with us.

It is an accomplishment and a journey etched in our minds forever.

Appendix: Where Do We Go from Here?

A woman loses her hearing at the age of 20 and is introduced to the solace of deafness. After years of being isolated--writing notes to communicate and living without music—she hunts for a solution and discovers the cochlear implant.

Yet another woman is active with two children and growing her husband's business when she has surgery for a spinal tumor, which leaves her with chronic pain. She eventually loses her job, begins living on assistance and closes the business. A friend introduces her to spinal cord stimulation and she is now back to being an active mom and working woman.

Just before his 53rd birthday, a pastor has his first seizure. Since then he experiences a decline in quality of life while taking anti-seizure medications; he can no longer maintain his active lifestyle. Frustrated with his decline, he is introduced to vagus nerve stimulation therapy. After receiving an implanted device, he gets weaned off all medications and is once again active in his church, and resumes cycling and other recreational activities.

A family goes on a ski vacation. After drinking contaminated water, the two teenage children develop delayed gastric emptying, or gastroparesis, and treatments are minimal. Formerly active children are now housebound. The mother looks for a solution meets the inventor of gastric electrical stimulation therapy. Both children get implanted with the devices, which were experimental at the time. Now, one is pursuing a Broadway career while the other is going to university. Both are now active young adults.

A veteran returns from the wars in Iraq and Afghanistan, but he doesn't return in the same condition that he departed. He now has locked-in syndrome due severe war injuries; his mind is fully functional but his body is completely paralyzed. His only means of communication is a series of eye blinks. Seeking a better quality of life for him, his wife finds a communication device that senses electrical signals from his facial muscles, which he uses to operate a computer. He now communicates with his family using the automated voice of the computer, sends and receives email messages, and plays video games with his son.

What do all these stories have in common? In each case a person with a disability or a caregiver hunting for an alternative therapy discover a neurotechnology solution to a serious neurological disease or disorder. Daily television advertisements and paid programming remind us of pharmaceutical options. But neurotechnology options seem to be discovered by those with good hunting skills. Granted, neurotechnology devices represent a relatively new frontier. But just as heart pacemakers have become more common, the notion of having an implanted neurotechnology device is becoming a more viable alternative for many people.

For people faced with chronic conditions, they are more commonly looking for alternative ways to find solutions than just taking the card that is handed to them. Many therapies and devices are available commercially in such areas as pain management, spasticity control, breathing assistance, and new rehabilitation techniques that are not necessarily integrated into common medical practice. Alternatively, participating in clinical trials requires careful consideration of the requisite time and financial commitments, along with a realistic consideration of expectations by the participant. There are exciting new technologies being investigated in research centers across the globe.

Promoting Awareness of Neurotechnology

At a National Institutes of Health Neural Prosthesis Workshop a few years back, a panel of neurotechnology users shared their experiences. The panel included a deaf person who had received a cochlear implant, a person with Parkinson's disease who had received a deep-brain stimulations system, a quadriplegic who had received an implanted hand grasp stimulator, and myself--a woman who had been implanted with an experimental standing prosthesis. Each of us reported that clinicians were sometimes hesitant to recommend the procedure because of reimbursement or other financial issues. In many cases, it was difficult to even find information on neurotechnology because the respective patient communities were not familiar with the changing technology. But after receiving our implants, each of us expressed extreme satisfaction with our devices and only regretted not opting in sooner.

Neurotech Network, an educational organization that I founded several years back, came from listening to stories like these and ones told earlier. Neurotech Network is a 501(c)(3) nonprofit organization dedicated to improving the education of and advocacy for access to neurotechnology for people with neurological impairments. Through the resources we have developed, we help people learn how these new alternative therapies and cutting-edge medical treatments impact the lives of people with neurological and psychiatric illnesses, diseases, and disabilities. These resources are available free from Neurotech Network. Visit www.NeurotechNetwork.org to review educational fact sheets, meet other people who use the technology, and search the only freely available online database of neurotechnology products.

All of this highlights the need for more awareness from clinical professionals and more understanding from the general public. It also points out one of the challenges confronting neurotechnology professionals in years ahead. We cannot expect funding agencies, investors, or clinicians to show a profound understanding if the public is still left in the dark.

Mom, Can We Keep It?

What happens to medical devices used in a clinical trial once the trial is complete? At the time of this writing, there are 130 active human clinical trials involving devices for neurological conditions in the U.S. For external devices, such as transcutaneous electric nerve stimulators (TENS) or surface muscle stimulators, the end of the clinical trial means handing the device back to the research team, in exchange for their appreciation for your services.

What about implanted devices?

For example, a person who participates in a multiyear clinical trial of a deep brain stimulation system may use the implanted device for a long period of time. During that time, the participant likely experiences life-changing results. Now, the research study has concluded. Research funding no longer covers long-term use or custodial care. Should the device be surgically removed? Some industry representatives suggest leaving the implanted device in the body but turning it off. In essence, it becomes medical garbage, not unlike the space junk left floating around in high earth orbit after various space initiatives were completed.

A long- standing misconception of research toward commercializing medical devices is that once a clinical trial is concluded and the study deemed successful, then the device will remain with the participant. Sadly, this is not the case. In fact, it is not the case even if the device is subsequently approved by the U.S. Food & Drug Administration (FDA). Just because a device has FDA approval does not mean that it is available to consumers. Once the commercialization process has run its course, the funding agencies have obtained their study results. The device industry has gleaned key selling points for the device. But what about the participant?

A participant in a research study should fully understand the risks associated with the clinical trial for a new device. A research study lasts for a finite period of time. Human research studies cannot exist without human participants. In the process, their rights are sometimes forgotten. More often than not, at the conclusion of a research study, medical garbage is left behind inside the bodies of human participants. There is no funding to continue to use the device if it is successful. If it is not successful, there may be no funding to explant the device, unless a life-threatening situation emerges. Further, there is a low perceived value to understanding long term use of devices. Is it right to give a person a better functioning life and then take it away in the name of scientific research?

There is no easy solution to the dilemma of what to do with medical devices at the conclusion of a research study. These post-trial scenarios are often an afterthought in research and development. This topic is the elephant in the room for the medical research and development community.

Although the study participant assumes the risk, the research and commercialization would not exist without human research participants. At some point, the device industry and research institutions will need to find a solution. It will only come when the interested parties work together to find it.

Who Pays for This Stuff?

Healthcare is expensive. It doesn't matter whether you think healthcare is a right or a privilege. Either way, it is expensive. Going over my medical bills after the accident gave me a rude awakening about what how much medical care can cost. Throw new technology into the mix and it becomes even more expensive. Our current funding system in the U.S. is a mix of private third-party payers and some publicly funded programs. Each has a different billing system and different means of evaluating what will be covered. Just because the FDA approves a new device or therapy as safe and effective, it does not mean there will be insurance coverage.

The neurotechnology industry, like the entire medical products industry, depends greatly on the outlook for health insurance reimbursement. And when it comes to reimbursement, there is no greater force than the U.S. Centers for Medicare and Medicaid Services (CMS). This agency's decisions and policies impact far more than the 40 million elderly and disabled Americans who participate in Medicare. Private insurers and state and foreign government agencies look to CMS for guidance on complex financial and technology issues. And both established healthcare firms and startups alike depend on CMS's coverage decisions as endorsement—or rebuke—for new procedures.

CMS has created a Council on Technology and Innovation,

comprised of a diverse group, which holds open forums for the public. I attended one of these forums recently and it was a real eye opener. The topic was an external electrical stimulation system therapy for treating people who have suffered a stroke. There were countless peer-reviewed journal articles about the therapy that demonstrated benefits. The device was also approved for reimbursement for incomplete spinal cord injury.

As it turned out, the forum that I attended was more of a "lobbying" process rather than a clinical meeting. There were many scientists, therapists, and industry representatives making the case for reimbursement. I understand the need to keep costs down, but the strategy of gaining coverage by lobbying leads to reimbursement only for the device firms with the deepest pockets.

The need for reimbursement is inherent in our health care system. Medical device companies need it as a revenue source and consumers need it to gain access to a new therapy. After my injury, I wrote countless appeal letters to my insurance company simply to gain access to rehabilitation technology involving electrical stimulation. This problem affects more than just those with spinal cord injury. A woman with multiple sclerosis was trying desperately to get access to a drop-foot stimulation system, but her insurance company consistently turned her down, claiming that a walking cane was more cost-effective.

The neurotechnology industry is taking notice of this. Many firms have reimbursement professionals (or bulldogs) whose sole function is to help submit insurance claims and help potential users make their case on appeal to denials. In the end, financial access is a war between quality of care and cost-containment with the consumer caught in the middle.

Fortunately, there have been some cases of creative thinking to find ways to provide access to new technologies. One case that comes to mind is FES cycling at acute care rehabilitation hospitals. FES cycles are an expensive piece of technology for a rehabilitation center. To help offer broader access, some rehabilitation centers are offering "gym memberships" to their facility after the patient has been discharged. This way the post-patient has access to the technology and the hospital has a continuing revenue stream to support the technology.

This is a first step to ease the barrier of financial access but it is only viable for external rehabilitation equipment. To apply the technique to implanted devices is simply impossible.

At the end of the day, we need to rethink how people with neurological conditions can gain access to proven technologies. Should it be just the chosen few or the population targeted in scientific studies?

www.ingramcontent.com/pod-product-compliance
Lightning Source LLC
LaVergne TN
LVHW010915110826
845149LV00013B/2371

* 9 7 8 0 9 8 8 2 3 4 2 0 8 *